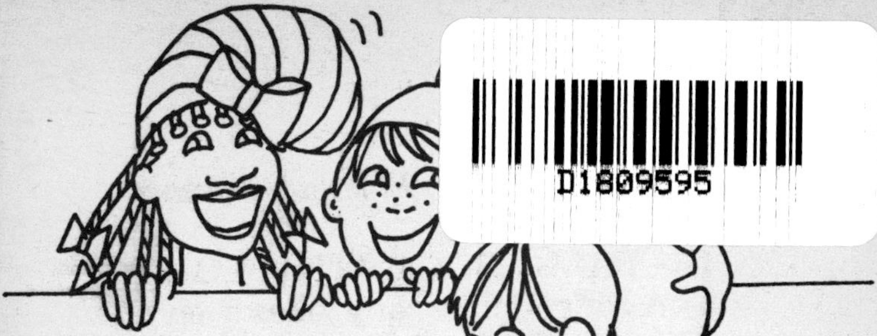

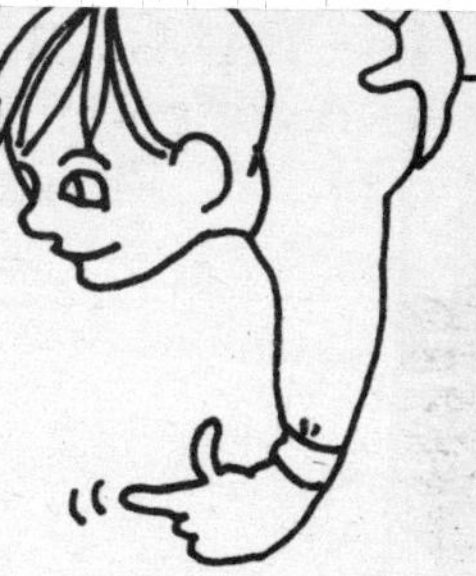

This copy of
**FLOELLA'S
FUNNIEST
JOKES**
belongs to

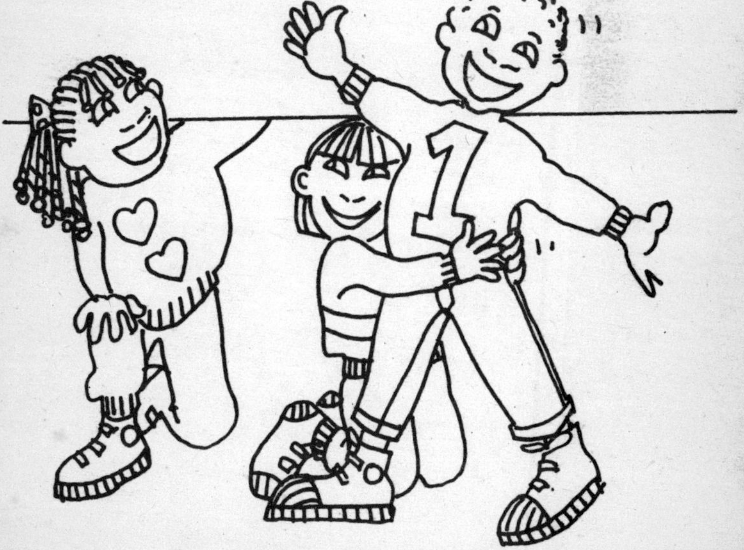

Also available by Floella Benjamin

FALL ABOUT WITH FLO
A collection of zany jokes from
Floella Benjamin

FLOELLA'S FUNNIEST JOKES

Floella Benjamin

Illustrated by Susan George

Beaver Books

A Beaver Book
Published by Arrow Books Limited
62–65 Chandos Place, London WC2N 4NW

An imprint of Century Hutchinson Ltd

London Melbourne Sydney Auckland
Johannesburg and agencies throughout the world

First published 1985

Text © Floella Benjamin 1985
Illustrations © Century Hutchinson Ltd 1985

Set in Century Schoolbook by
JH Graphics Limited, Reading

Made and printed in Great Britain
by Anchor Brendon Ltd
Tiptree, Essex

ISBN 09 943120 3

To Nicola and Taron

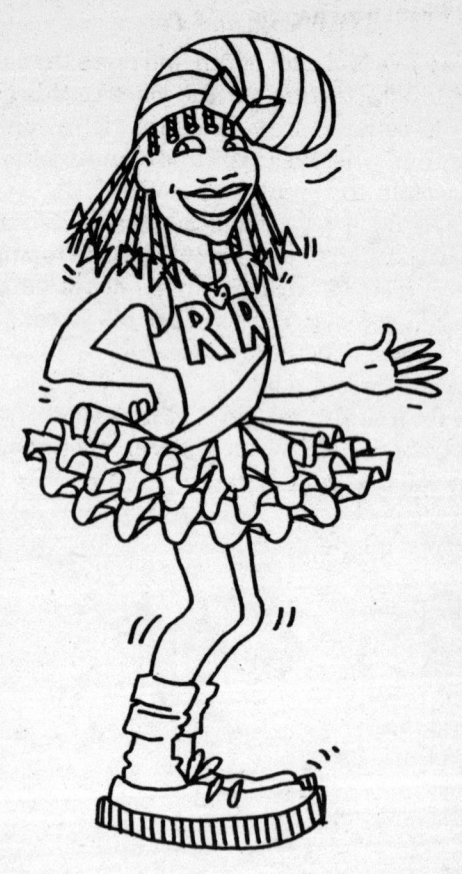

A Word From Floella ...

I must say I've had a lot of fun and more than my fair share of laughs testing out the jokes in this book on people. I believe that laughter is a universal language and wherever I go I find a funny joke always relaxes people and breaks the ice.

My son Aston loves telling jokes and he made up several of the ones in this book. He's developing quite a sense of humour which will no doubt be a great asset as he grows up. Here's one of his jokes:

'Doctor! Doctor! I feel like a radiator.'

'Mmmm you do look a bit hot.'

Not bad for a three year old . . . thanks son.

Oh and I'd better not forget to thank my hubby Keith and his Macintosh computer for helping me to compile the book.

Have a good giggle.

Love Floella

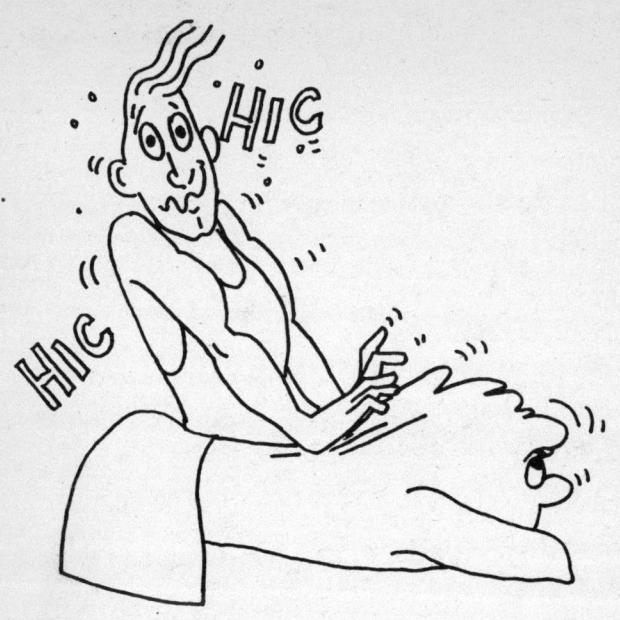

What do you get if you cross a bottle of liver salts and a masseuse?
A fizzy o therapist.

What do a toucan, a pelican and a taxman have in common?
They all have big bills.

What do you call a woman with a piano keyboard on her head?
Joanna.

What do you call a man who's always around
when you need him?
Andy.

What do you call a man who gets up your
nose?
Vic.

Did you hear about the wally who went on a
crash diet?
He wrecked three cars and a bus.

What do you call a man who lies on the floor?
Matt.

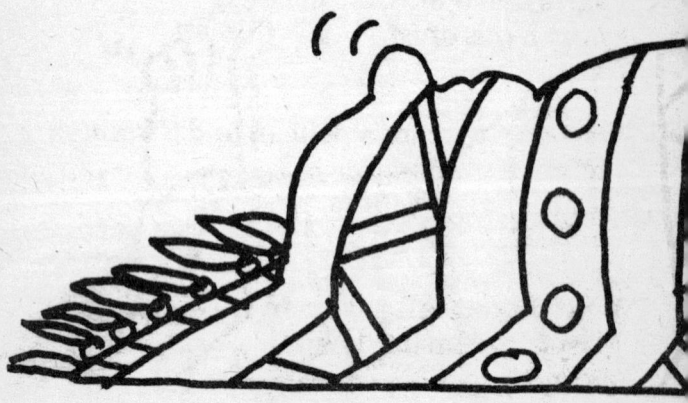

What do you call two burglars?
A pair of knickers.

What do you call a deer with no eyes?
No idea.

What do you call a man with a bee on his toe?
Toby.

Why do cowboys ride into town?
'Cos they're too heavy to carry.

WALLY: Does this train run on time?
GUARD: *No it runs on tracks.*

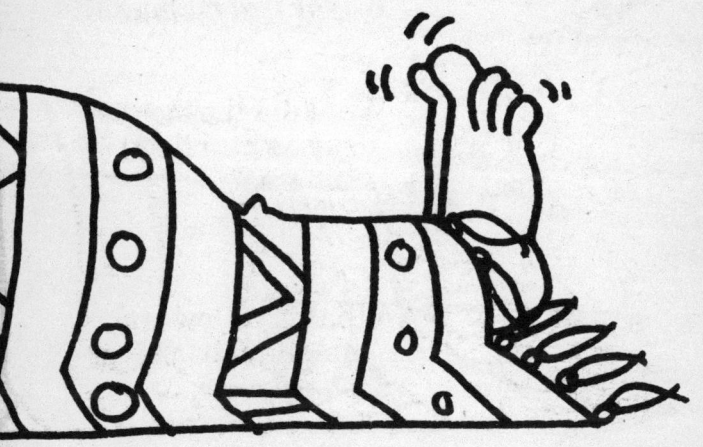

Did you here about the wally who ate a sofa
and two chairs?
He had a (suite) tooth.

What do you call a woman who's afraid of
textile factories?
Mildred.

'Doctor! Doctor! Yesterday I felt like a
marquee and today I feel like a bell tent.'
*'Mmm I know what's wrong with you. You're
too tense.'*

Knock, Knock.
Who's there?
Wayne.
Wayne who?
Wayne in a manger . . .

What did the monkey
say as he fell out of
the tree?
ARGGH!

What is yellow and
smells of bananas?
Monkey puke.

BOSS: Hey Wally, did you post that wig off to the customer?
WALLY: *Yes Boss, I sent it hair mail.*

What is Nelson's baby brother called?
Half-Nelson.

What do you get if you cross a French emperor with a ton of TNT?
Napolean Blownapart.

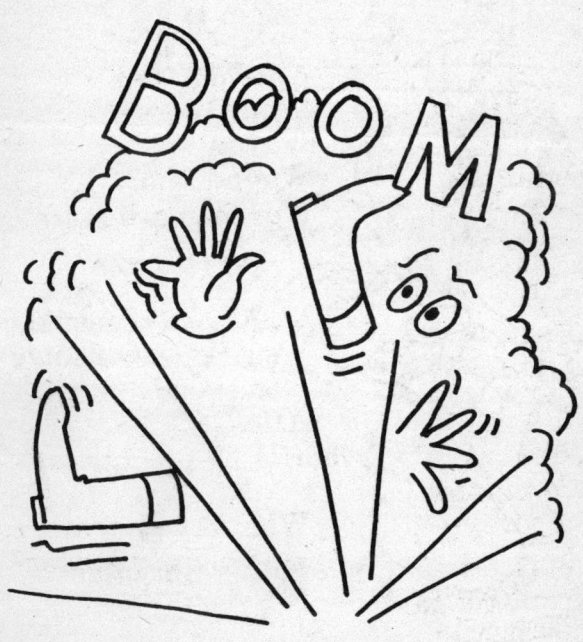

What do you call a man with lovely trees and
  flowers and a pretty little pond on his
  head?
Dell

What is a specimen?
An Italian astronaut.

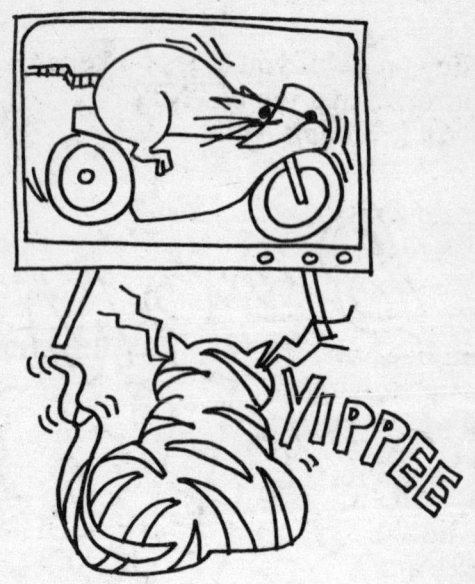

What is a cat's favourite TV programme?
Miami Mice.

What nationality is Father Christmas?
North Polish.

How do you know Father Christmas loves
gardening?
He's always going hoe, hoe, hoe.

Why does a dog bark?
'Cos if he miaowed he'd be a cat.

What are eggshells used for?
To keep eggs together.

Where do wallys go to school?
A Wally-technic.

Did you hear about the wally who ran a
two-minute mile?
He found a short cut.

What did the Pink Panther say when he trod
on the ant?
*Dead ant . . . dead ant, dead ant dead ant
dead ant.*

Which is the naughtiest superhero?
Bratman.

TEACHER: What's the fastest member of the cat family?
WALLY: *An E-type Jaguar?*

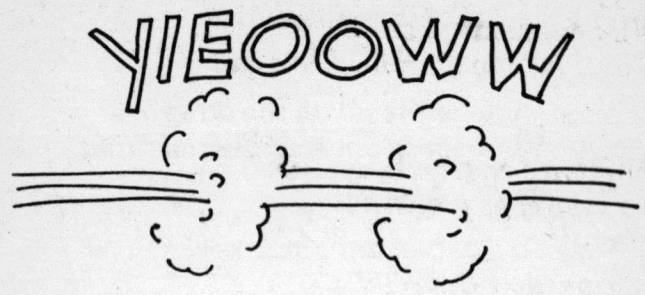

What kind of car does action man drive?
A <u>Toy</u>ota.

How did Moses divide the Red Sea?
With see-saw.

What do you call two pigs who live together?
Pen friends.

Did you hear about the wally farmer who planted rows and rows of gramophone records?
He was trying to grow popcorn.

How do chickens start a race?
From scratch.

What did the rabbit do when he grew up?
He joined the Hare Force.

What did one lift say to the other?
I think I'm going down with something.

Why do giraffes have long necks?
'Cos their feet smell.

What lies on the ground a hundred feet up?
A centipede on its back.

What do you get if you cross an American
president with a shark?
Jaws Washington.

What do you call an underground train full
of professors?
A tube of Smarties.

What does Bugs Bunny use when he goes
fishing?
A hare net.

How many seconds in a year?
Twelve . . . the 2nd Jan, the 2nd Feb . . . etc.

Why did the bank robber take a bath?
So he could make a clean getaway.

Why did the angel lose his job?
'Cos he had harp failure.

What kind of driver never gets arrested?
A screwdriver.

This goldfish you sold me is always asleep.
That's not a goldfish it's a kipper.

What do you call a man who's black and blue
    all over?
Bruce.

Did you hear about the wally who tried to
get a job as a cameraman at Radio One?

SNAKE BREEDING by Anna Conda.

What do you get if you drop a piano on a
soldier?
A flat major.

Knock, Knock.
Who's there?
Debbie.
Debbie who?
Debbie a welcome in the hillside.

What time do Chinamen go to the dentist?
Tooth hurtie

Knock, Knock.
Who's there?
A dun up.
A dun up who?
*Oooo you smelly
    thing.*

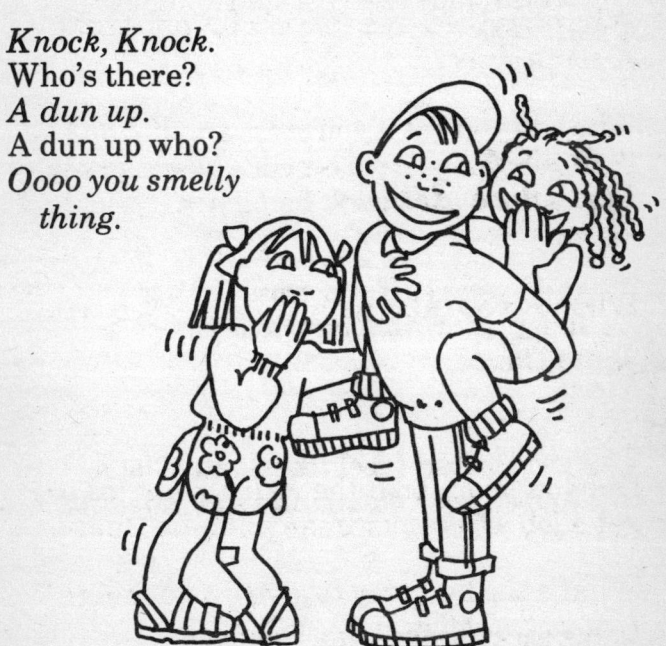

What's green and smells?
Kermit's nose.

Did you hear about the wally who was
     teaching his dog to wee in the gutter?
He fell off the roof.

Did you hear about the man with five legs?
His trousers fit him like a glove.

What animal is really stupid and hums?
A wally bee.

What do you get if you cross an idiot and a
     climber?
The wally and the ivy.

What do you get if you cross Father
     Christmas with a ferocious tiger?
Santa Claws.

'Doctor! Doctor! I feel like Santa Claus.'
'Well, open your mouth and say "ho ho ho".'

What's the best way to give up smoking?
Use wet matches.

WALLY: *If you put your tooth under your pillow, a big ship will come and take it away.*

WALLY'S FRIEND: A big ship?

WALLY: *Yes, it's called the Tooth Ferry.*

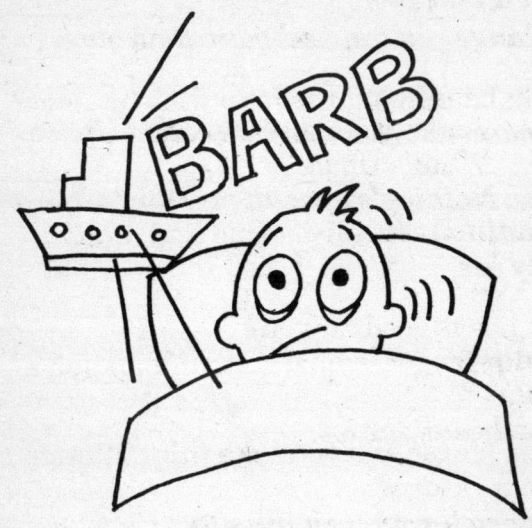

Did you hear about the wally who got travel sickness just by licking an airmail stamp?

My Dad's nose is so big he only has to breathe in once and it lasts him all day.

Sign outside the Tax Office: SORRY – WE'RE OPEN.

What do you call a man with some drums on his head.
Kit.

What do you get if you cross an orange with a bell?
An orange you can peel more than once.

DOCTOR: *You've got a disease called Updoc.*
PATIENT: What's Updoc?
DOCTOR: *Nothing's up with me. You're the one who's ill.*

What bee is good for you?
Vitamin B.

DOCTOR: Nurse, did you take this patient's temperature?
NURSE: *No Doctor, is it missing?*

DOCTOR: Quickly give this patient artificial respiration!
PATIENT: *Just a minute I'm a private patient. I want the real thing!*

How do you fix a leaking airship?
With Helium.

What does Father Christmas
    get if he is
    stuck in a chimney?
Santa Claustrophobia.

What is small, has
    pointed ears and is a
    great detective?
Sherlock Gnomes.

What do you call a
    woman in church
    spire?
Belle.

'Doctor! Doctor! I've
    got a terrible
    memory.'
*'Well in that case,
    would you mind
    paying in advance!'*

What's soft and white
    and comes from outer
    space?
A martian mellow.

What do climbers eat
    for tea?
Rock cakes.

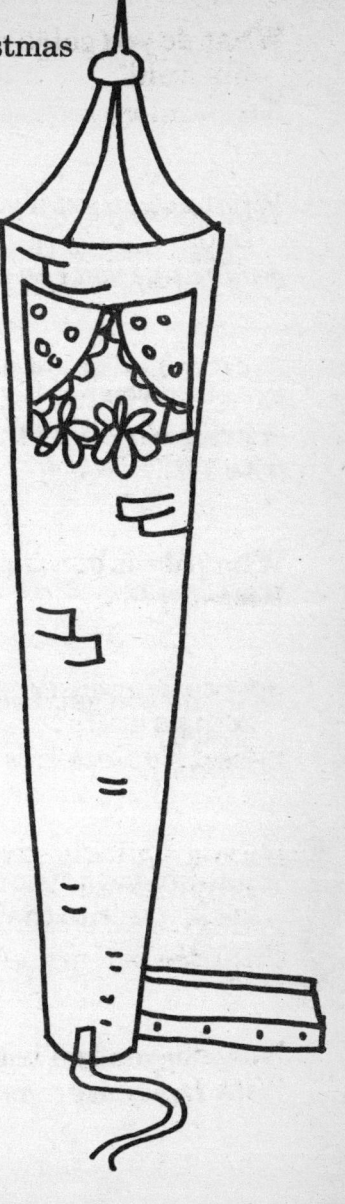

What do you get if you cross a dog with a test-tube?
A laboratory retriever.

What do you get if you cross a seven-foot-tall green man with a fountain pen?
The Ink-credible Hulk.

What do you get if you cross a Mercedes, a dog and a broom?
A car-pet-sweeper.

Where do climbers go in the evenings?
Rock concerts.

What do you get if you cross a padlock with a shark?
Lockjaws.

What kind of music do you get if you throw a rock star into the lake?
New Wave.

'Why do you call your car Bunny?'
''Cos I only use it for short hops.'

What do you get if you cross a cockerel and a
    clock?
An alarm cluck.

What do you get if you cross a soldier with a
    parrot?
A parrotrooper.

What do you get if you cross a clown with a
    spiritualist?
A happy medium.

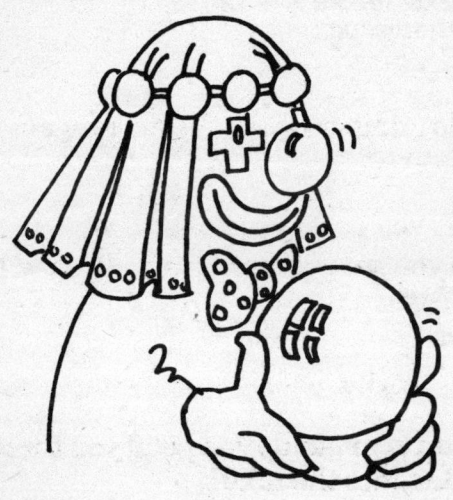

What do you get if you cross a parrot and a
    bee?
*A bird that's always telling you how busy it
is.*

What do you get if you cross a sick eagle with a robber?
An illegal ill eagle.

What do you get if you replace a wally's brain with an elastic band?
A real stretch of the imagination.

WALLY: Teacher, how long can someone live without a brain?
TEACHER: *How old are you?*

What tells jokes and lays eggs?
A comedi-hen.

What do you get if you cross a potato with a computer?
Micro chips.

TEACHER: Wally, why are you using a pocket calculator?
WALLY: *To add up how many pockets I've got, Miss.*

What do they serve for lunch in the canteens at nuclear power stations?
Fission Chips.

What colour is the wind?
Blew.

'Doctor! Doctor! I'm so indecisive.'
Mmm, have you got a headache?
Well, yes and no . . .

Where do kings go to buy their homes?
Newcastle.

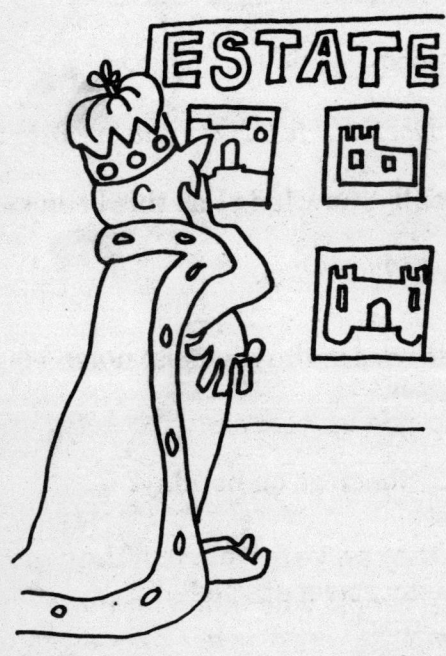

What is green and red and spins round at a
   hundred miles an hour?
Kermit in a blender.

Where do spiders live?
Crawley.

Where is the best place to buy eggs?
Henley.

What kind of car do dogs like best?
A Rover.

'Doctor! Doctor! I feel like I can see into the
   future.'
'Mmm really, how long has this been going
   on?'
'Since next Thursday.'

Where do cars make the most noise?
Tooting.

Where do sheep go on holiday?
Ramsgate.

Where do people who talk a lot live?
Chatham.

What do you get if you cross a skinhead with a lawnmower?
A bovver mower.

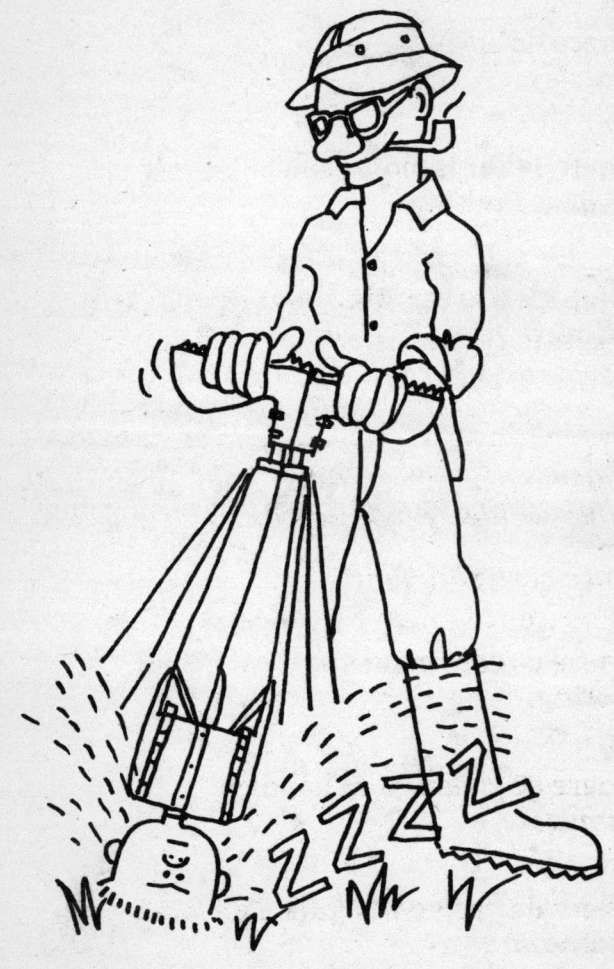

'Doctor! Doctor! I feel like a pack of cards.'
'Wait here . . . I'll deal with you later.'

How did you get a puncture Wally?
I think there was a fork in the road.

What ballet is most popular with frogs?
Swamp lake.

What do you get if you cross a duck with a genius?
A wise quacker.

Did you hear about Wally's new invention?
Double-sided playing cards.

Where do pigs leave their cars?
Porking meters.

Why can't a bike stand up?
'Cos it's too tired.

What's JR's favourite sweet?
Ewing gum.

What do you call a girl with a picture of the
    Queen stamped on the side of her head?
Penny.

Where is Solomon's temple?
On the side of his head.

What do you call a girl with a frog on her
    head?
Lily.

What do you call a man
    sitting on the side of
    the M1 about thirty
    miles from
    Birmingham?
Lester.

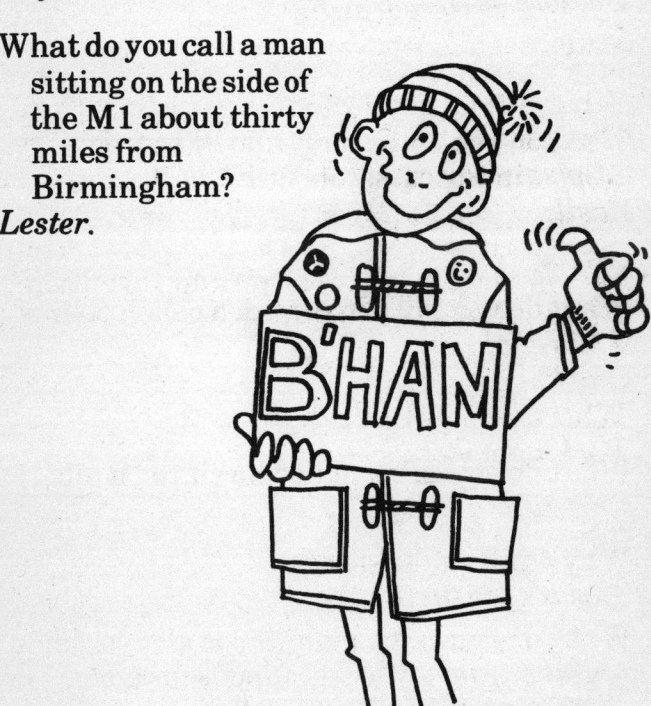

What do you call a Spaniard whose car has
    been stolen?
Carlos.

What do you call a man lying in the gutter?
Dwayne.

What do you call a man who keeps getting
    into a casserole dish.
Stew.

What do you call a man who likes to join
    Stew in the casserole dish?
Basil.

What do you call a man with a pencil behind
    his ear?
Clark.

What do you call a man who sits on a pile of
    wood?
Guy.

What do you call a man who is always being
    given away by local councils for home
    improvements?
Grant.

What's the closest thing to silver?
The Lone Ranger's bum.

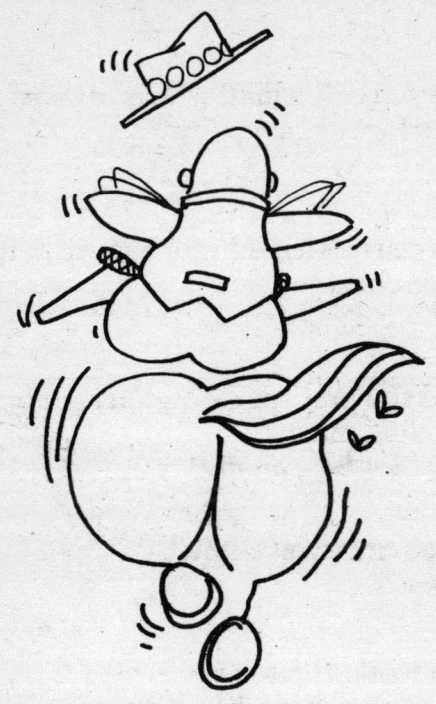

What do you call a man who is eight feet tall
   with a pointed head?
Lance.

What do you call a girl who sits on bars in
   cocktail lounges?
Olive.

What do you call a man who is overdrawn at the bank?
Owen.

What do you call a man who is covered from head to foot in gold paint?
Oscar.

What do you call a man who has red paint all over his chest?
Robin.

What did the first smoke signal sent by a Red Indian mean?
'Help my blanket's on fire!'

What tree can't you climb?
A lavatory.

Why is a football pitch wet?
'Cos the players keep dribbling on it.

Why can't you find aspirins in the jungle?
'Cos the parrots eat'em all.

What do you call a girl who's covered in chocolate?
Candy.

What do you call a girl who keeps getting
    thrown overboard?
Annette.

What do you call a girl who is always in the
    bookies?
Betty.

What do you call a girl with a three course
    lunch on her head?
Dinah.

What do you call a girl who always arrives
    before dinner?
Grace.

What do you call a girl who can pull the
    roof off a house?
Gail.

What do you do
    if your nose
    goes on strike?
Pick it.

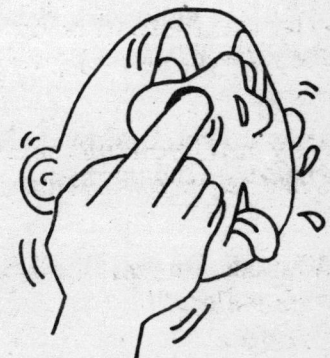

What do you call a girl who is stuck down a
  drain?
Ingrid.

What do you call a Spanish lady with one
  tooth?
Oneta.

Who shouted 'Knickers' at the big bad wolf?
Little Rude Riding Hood.

How do you get an ant out of your ear?
*Pour chocolate down it and it will come out a
  treat.*

What's green inside and white outside?
A frog sandwich.

What do you call a chicken's ghost?
A poultrygist.

How do you make a jacket last?
Make the trousers first.

TEACHER: Do you like Dickens?
WALLY: *I don't know, miss, I've never been
  there.*

Where do cows go on holiday?
Moo York.

'Doctor! Doctor! How can I stop this cold
   Going to my chest?'
'Tie a knot in your neck.'

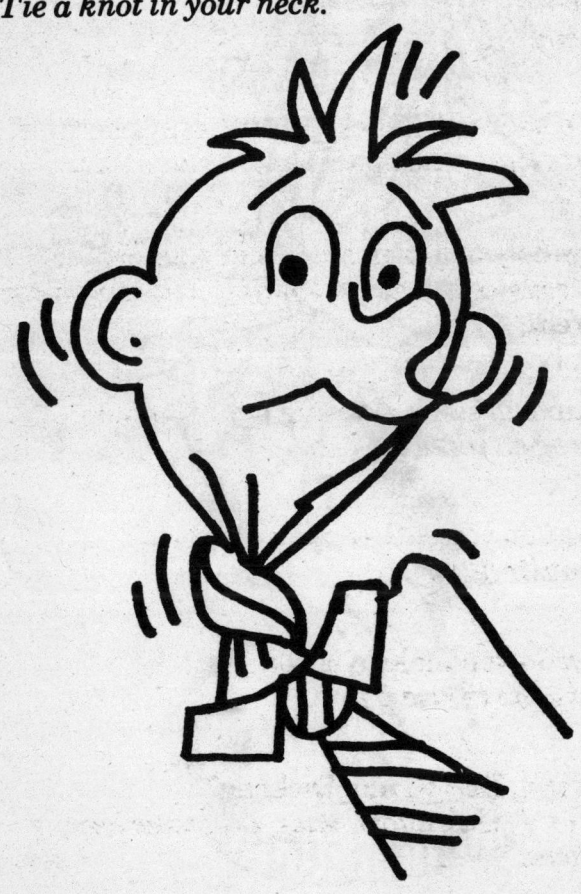

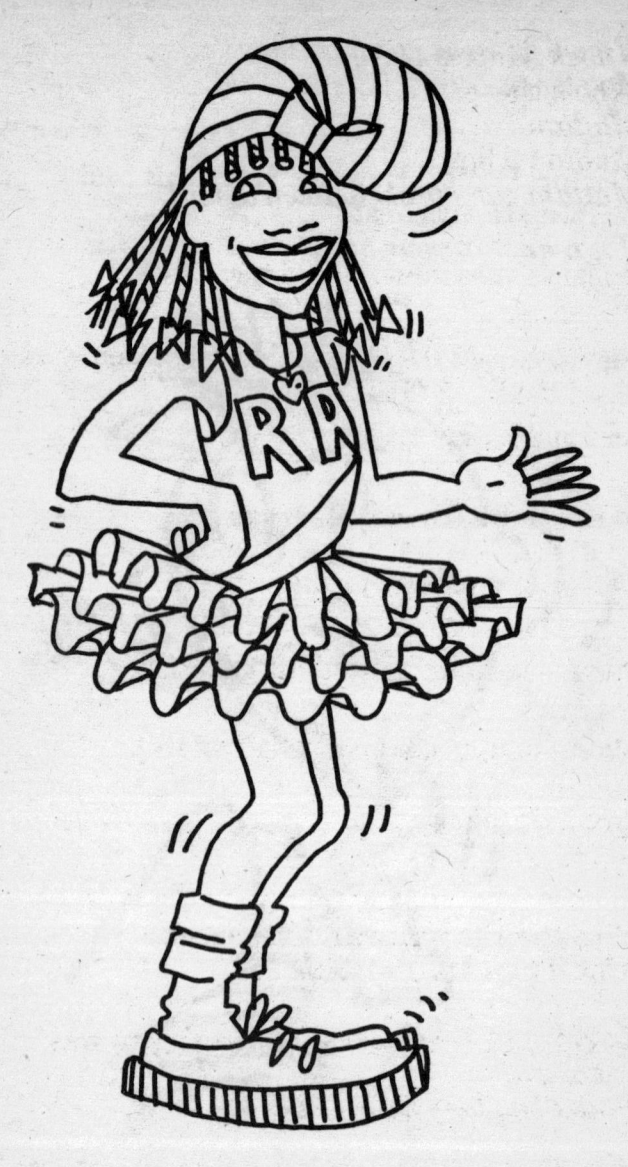

Knock, Knock.
Who's there?
Madam.
Madam who?
Madam car's broken down outside.

EMBARRASSING MOMENTS by Lucy Lastic.

HOW I OVERCAME SHYNESS by M. Barrassed.

SLIMMING by Di. Ette.

WOOD CARVING by Ray Zer Sharp.

SLEEPLESS NIGHTS by Lisa Wake.

THE SMASH AND GRAB by Chukka Brick.

CHOOSING THE BEST MEAT by Selena Cut.

Where's Felixtowe?
On the end of his foot.

Why did the wally eat ten pence?
'Cos it was his dinner money.

Last night a police dog-handler's van was
    stolen.
Police say they have no leads.

Why do golfers carry an extra sock?
In case they get a hole in one.

'Hey, why did you buy a black and white dog Wally?'
''Cos the licence is cheaper.'

'Hey Wally, why did you put that fish in your piano?'
''Cos it's a piano-tuna.'

Where do frogs with bad eyesight go?
An hoptician.

What did the carpet say to the floor?
'OK kid, I've got you covered.'

'Waiter, there's a brick in my food!'
'Well, it is cottage pie, Sir.'

Knock, Knock.
Who's there?
Ivor.
Ivor who?
Ivor sore hand from knocking.

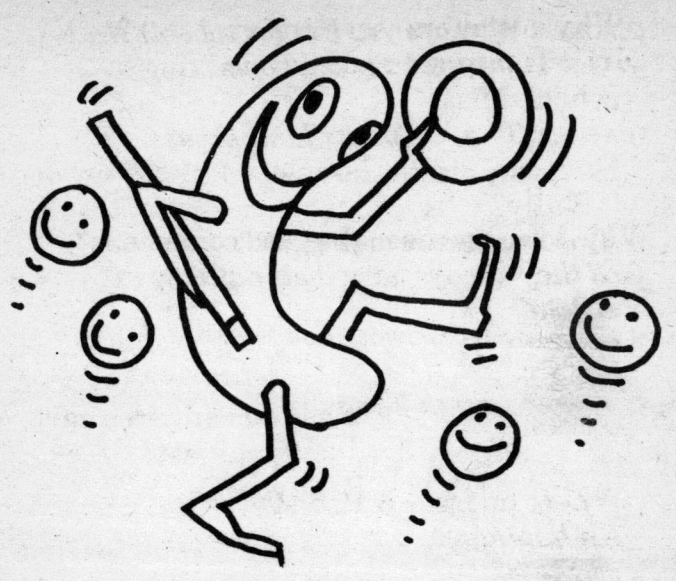

TEACHER: Why are you laughing at your
school dinner, Wally?
WALLY: *'Cos it looks funny, Miss.*

What do you get if you dial
75839875645367332691?
A sore finger.

'Hey Wally, how do you make a bandstand?'
'Take their chairs away?'

TEACHER: *Why are you late for school, Wally?*
WALLY: I sprained my ankle walking to school, Miss.
TEACHER: *That's a pretty lame excuse.*

Why do surgeons make good comediens?
'Cos they always have their patients in stitches.

What do vampires have for breakfast?
Readyneck.

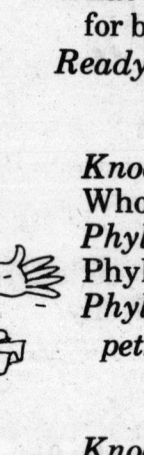

Knock, Knock.
Who's there?
Phyllis.
Phyllis who?
Phyllis car up with petrol please.

Knock, Knock.
Who's there?
Sal.
Sal who?
Salong way to Tipperary . . .

Knock, Knock.
Who's there?
Toby.
Toby who?
Toby or not Toby, that is the question . . .

Knock, Knock.
Who's there?
Aardvark.
Aardvark who?
*Aardvark a million miles for one of your
    smiles.*

'Waiter, this steak is so tough I can't cut it!'
*'Just a moment, Sir, I'll get you a sharper
    knife.'*

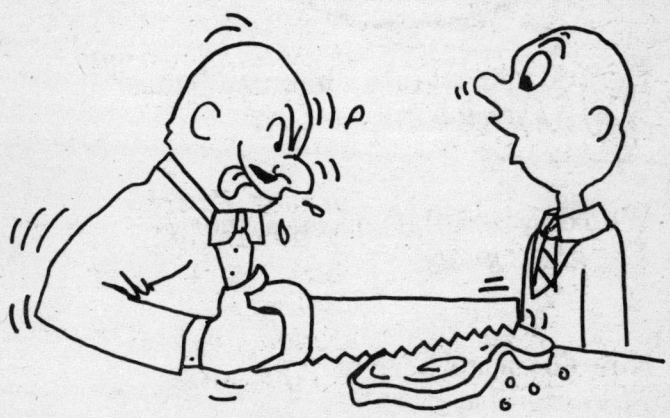

'My budgie died of 'flu.'
'Budgies don't get 'flu.'
'Mine flew into an electric fan.'

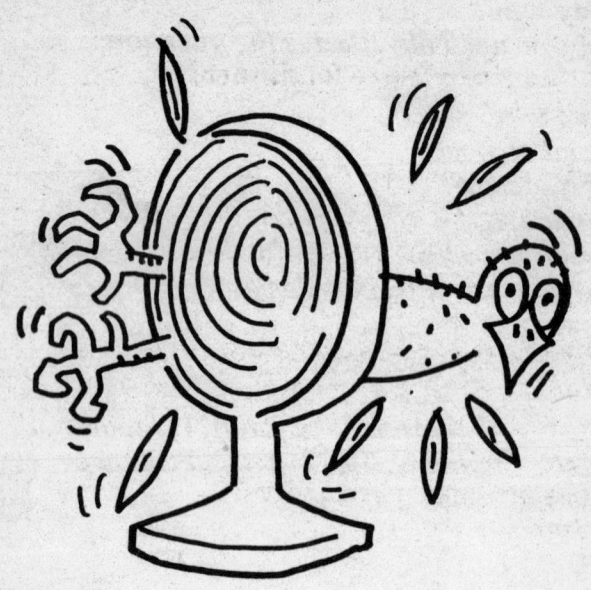

How do you get into a haunted house?
With a skeleton key.

Who do you call if you see a ghost?
The ghost guard.

How do ghosts keep fit?
They exorcise.

How do you check whether a house is
   haunted?
Use a spirit level.

What do ghosts have for dinner?
Ghoulash.

'Is your dad an artist, Wally?'
'Well, he's been drawing the dole for years.'

Where do theatre people live?
Acton.

Where do darts' players live?
Dartmoor.

Where is the best place to leave England?
Exeter.

MY GOLDEN WEDDING by Annie Versary.

A HUNDRED GOOD EXCUSES by Misty Bus.

MAKE A PROFIT by Maxie Mumgain.

THE LEANING TOWER OF PISA
by Selena Thataway.

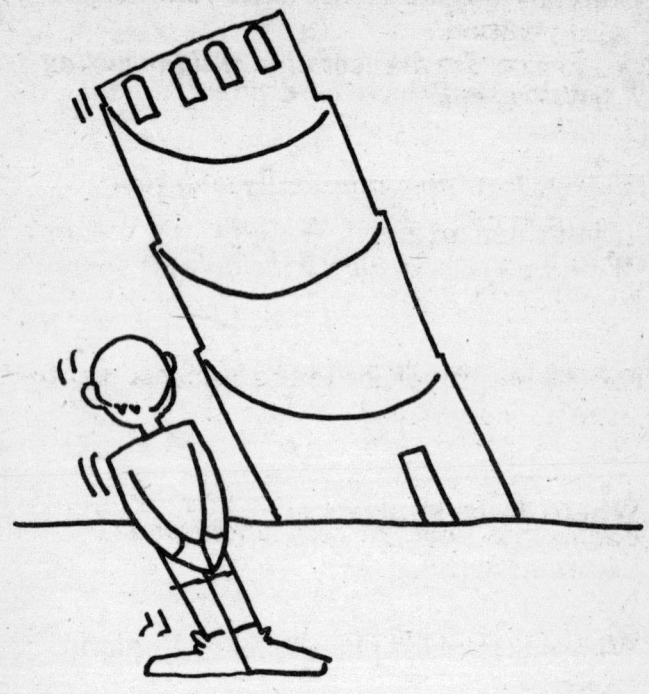

DOWN AND OUT by Len Duzaquid.

HOUSEHOLD ACCIDENTS by Luke Out.

TEACHER: How come you don't know the answer, Wally?
WALLY: *Well, if I knew the answer I wouldn't need to come here, Miss!*

WALLY PILOT: *This is flight 123 requesting permission to land.*

FLIGHT CONTROLLER: Please state your height and position.

WALLY PILOT: *I'm five foot nine and I'm sitting in the cockpit!*

'Did you hear about the wally who kept saying no?'
'No.'
'So you're the wally...

'Excuse me, do you know the quickest way to the police station?'
'Yea – run.'

'Excuse me, have you seen a policeman around here?'
'No.'
'Good ... stick 'em up!'

'Did you hear about the wally going to the mind-reader?'
'No, what happened?'
'He got his money back.'

What did the long hosepipe say to the short hosepipe?
'You little squirt.'

I wouldn't say Wally was mean but he does keep a fork in the sugar bowl.

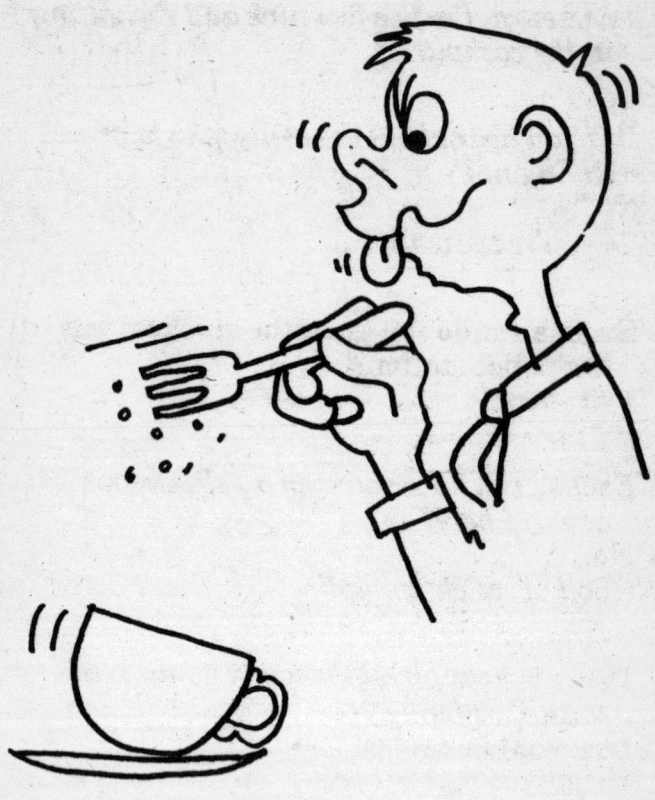

'Mummy do you notice any change in me?'
'No Dear, why do you ask?'
'I've just swallowed my pocket money!'

'Doctor! Doctor! I've just swallowed a pencil!'
'Well sit down and write your name.'

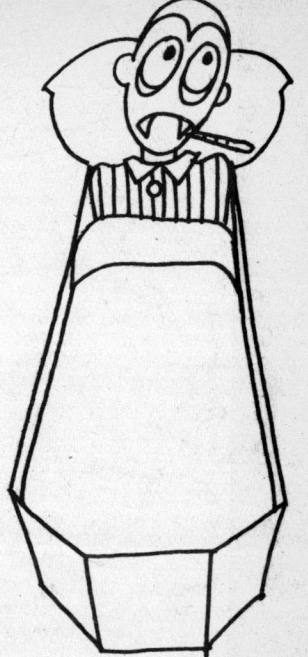

What does Dracula take when he has 'flu?
Coffin drops.

GAMEKEEPER: Hey, you can't fish there!
POACHER: *I know, I ain't caught a thing all day!*

'Waiter, I've just found this button in my dinner!'
'*Mmmm it must have fallen off the jacket potato.*'

What grows in the garden and is a Kung-Fu expert?
Bruce Leek.

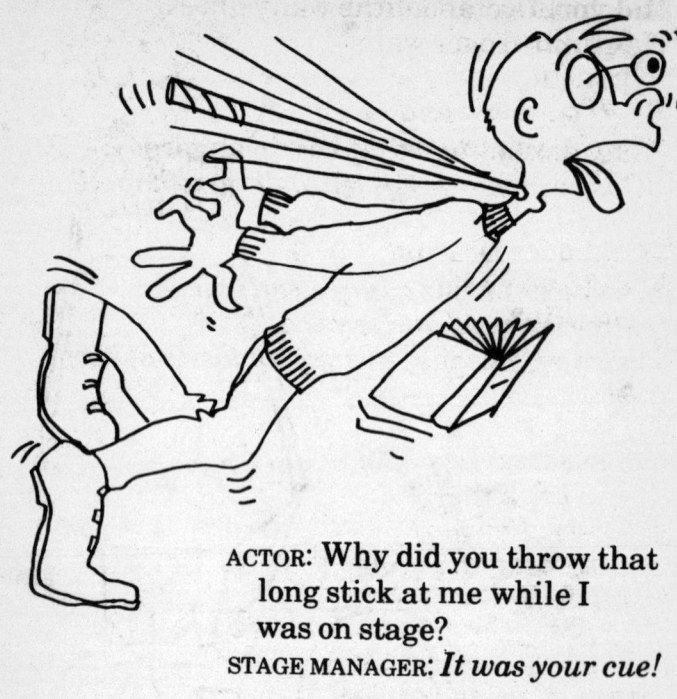

ACTOR: Why did you throw that long stick at me while I was on stage?
STAGE MANAGER: *It was your cue!*

Wally has decided to become a stunt man. He's going to jump over twenty motorbikes in a double-decker bus.

CUSTOMER: *You told me this watch was shockproof, waterproof and automatic.*
SHOPKEEPER: It is, Sir. What's the problem?
CUSTOMER: *It caught fire!*

Did you hear about the wally ghost?
He climbed over walls.

'Why do they call that boy "Kangaroo"?'
''Cos every one keeps telling him to hop it!'

CUSTOMER: *This is a very clean cafe.*
WAITER: Why do you say that?
CUSTOMER: *Because everything tastes of soap!*

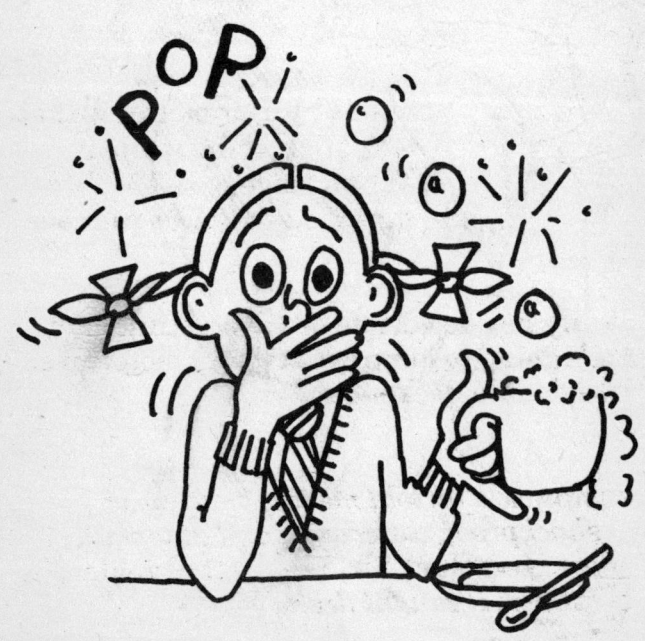

Think of a number and close your eyes . . .
Dark isn't it!

TEACHER: Out of a hundred apples, Jimmy
   gave Tommy six, Lucy four and ate fifteen
   himself. What was Jimmy left with?
WALLY: *Indigestion!*

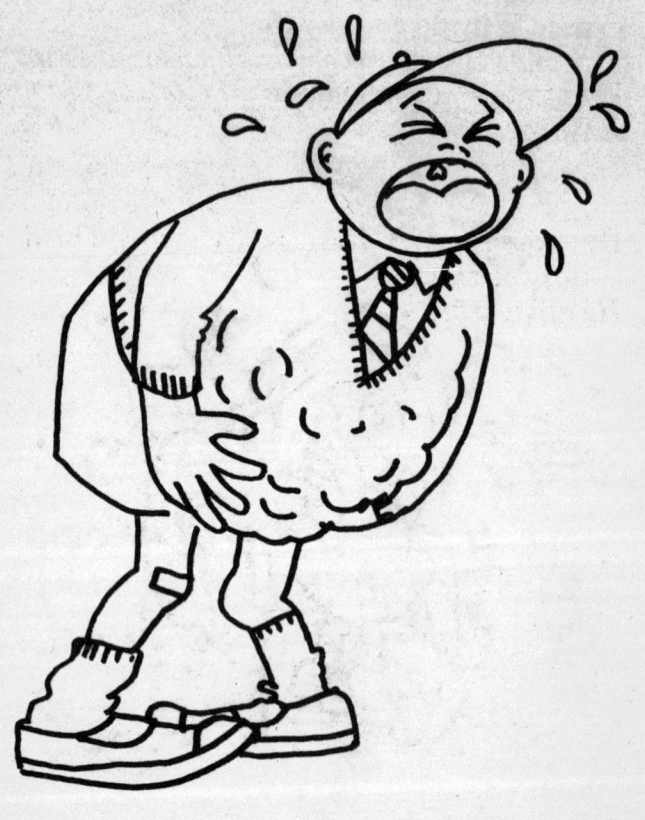

A teddy boy was working on a demolition site. One day, someone stole his pick axe so he went to report it to the boss.

'Don't worry,' said the boss, 'today's the day the teddy boys have their picks nicked!'

TEACHER: Any questions?
WALLY: *Yes Miss, when are you going?*

What goes 'cloak, cloak'?
A Chinese frog.

Did you hear about the wally who did bird impressions?
He ate worms.

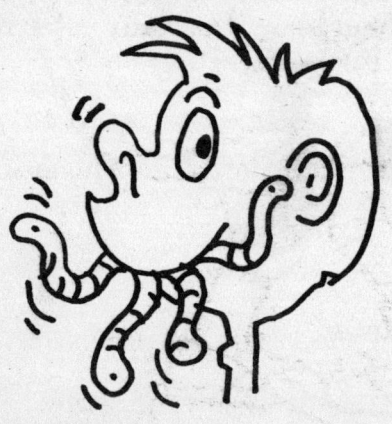

What soap powder do pilots use?
Ariel.

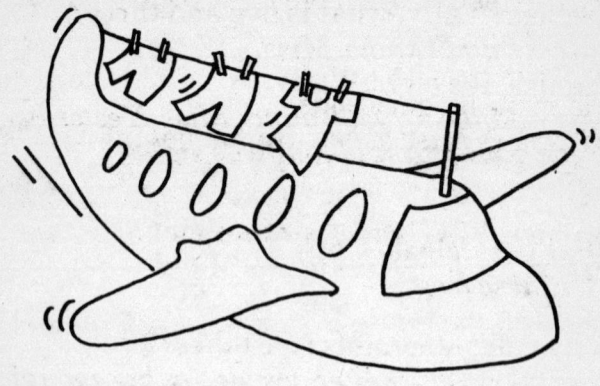

Did you hear about the wally caterpillar?
It turned into a frog.

What do you call an Eskimo's house that has
no toilet?
An Ig.

TEACHER: *Wally, name two pronouns.*
WALLY: Who me?
TEACHER: Correct. WELL DONE!

TEACHER: Eight, nine, ten. What comes next, Wally?

WALLY: *Er . . . Jack, Queen, King, Miss.*

TEACHER: Wally, what is five and three?

WALLY: *I don't know, Miss.*

TEACHER: It's eight Wally.

WALLY: *Make up your mind, Miss. Yesterday you said four and four was eight.*

TEACHER: Who invented the phone?

WALLY: *Er, the Phoenicians Miss?*

Why can't elephants ride bikes?
'Cos they don't make bicycle clips big enough.

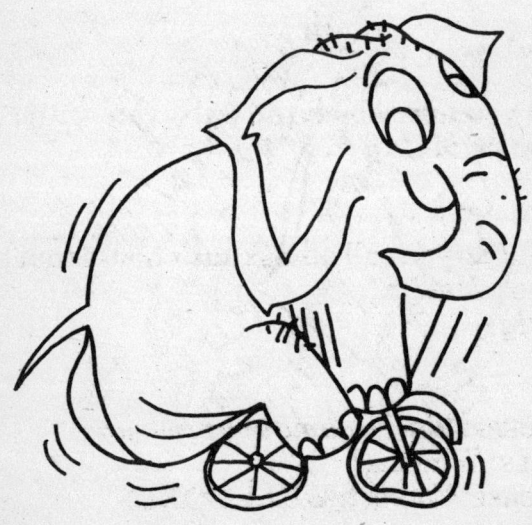

TEACHER: What's the longest sentence you can think of, Wally?
WALLY: *Er, life imprisonment, Miss.*

'Hey Wally, what do you run a hundred metres in?'
'Er ... a tee shirt, shorts and running shoes.'

Wally sent his photograph to the Lonely Hearts Club.
They sent it back saying they weren't that lonely.

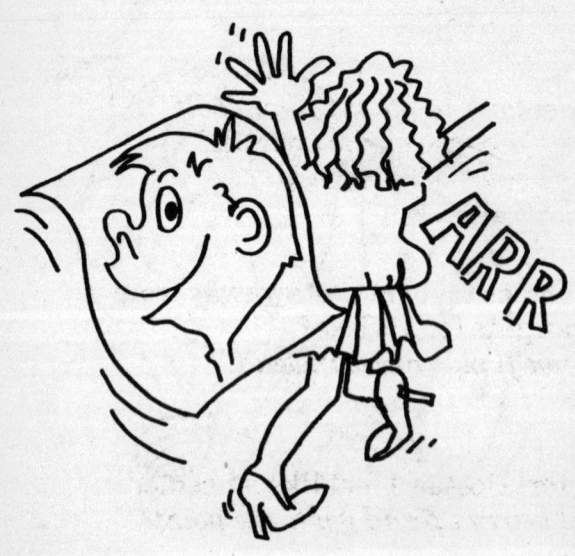

'Are we poisonous?' the young snake asked
    his dad.
'Yes we are, son,' replied his dad, 'why do you
    ask?'
''Cos I've just bitten my tongue.'

'I'm going to marry the boy next door,' said
    little Wallena to her friend.
'Oh really why is that?'
''Cos I'm not allowed to cross the road.'

'Hey Wally, what are you going to be *if* you
    grow up?'

'My doctor told me to give up golf.'
'Why – because of your health?'
'No, he saw my score card!'

'My doctor told me to stay away from
    draughts for a while.'
'OK, we'll play chess instead.'

'Doctor! Doctor! I feel like a needle.'
'Well hurry up and get to the point.'

'Doctor! Doctor! I've swallowed my mouth
   organ!'
'It's a good job you weren't playing the
   saxaphone!'

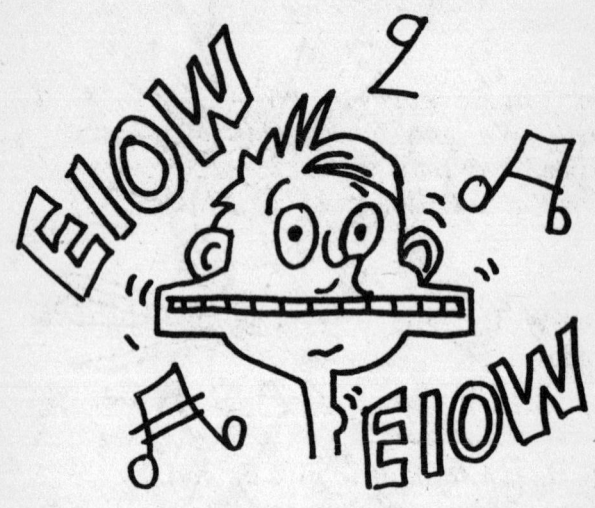

What stays hot in the fridge?
Mustard.

Boy and girl at the cinema.
BOY: *Comfortable?*
GIRL: Yes thanks.
BOY: *Can you see OK?*
GIRL: Yes thanks.
BOY: *Well would you mind swapping seats?*

'What has seventeen letters, begins with 'A',
ends with 'G' and means incredible pain?
'ARRRRRHHHHHHHHHG!'

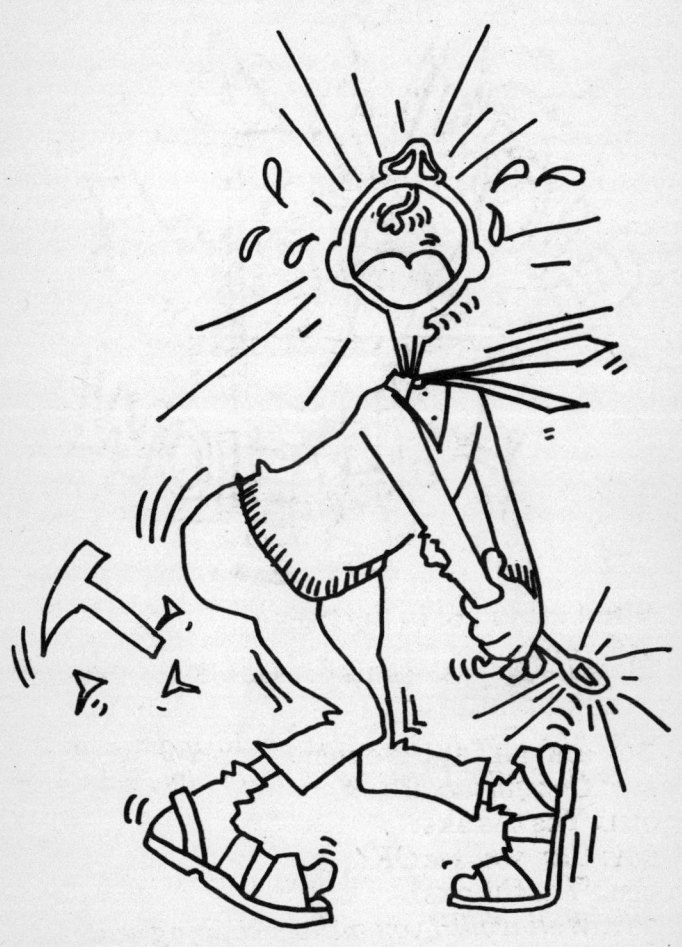

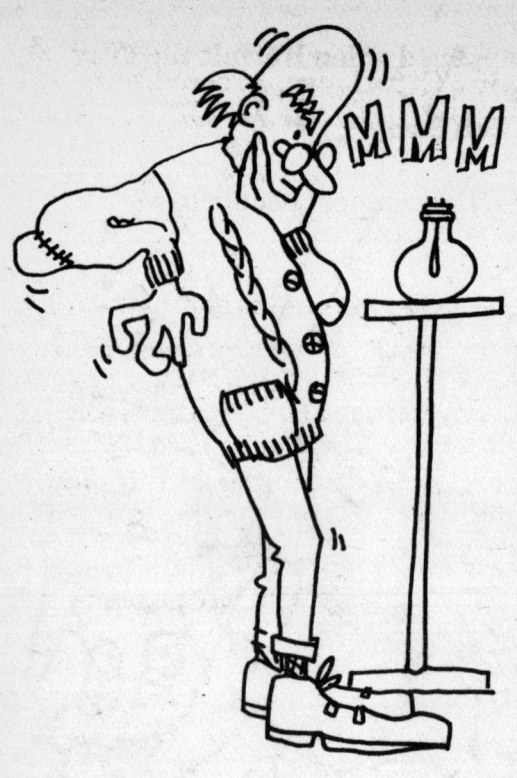

How many historians does it take to change
a light bulb?
*Twenty! One to change the bulb and nineteen
to talk about how good the old one was.*

Which Arab invented flavoured crisps?
Sultan vinegar.

What happened when Kermit the Frog
   parked on a yellow line?
He was toad away.

Where do the cleanest people live?
Bath.

Where do sea captains go to get their sailors?
Crewe.

BARMAN: Why is your dog wearing black
   shoes?
CUSTOMER: *'Cos his brown ones are at the
   menders.*

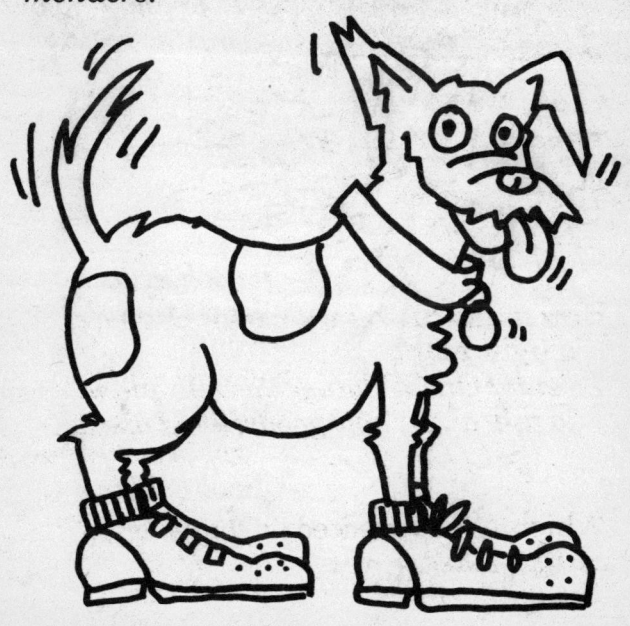

Knock, Knock.
Who's there?
Soup.
Soup who?
Souperman.

Knock, Knock.
Who's there?
Juno.
Juno who?
*Juno what time
 it is?*

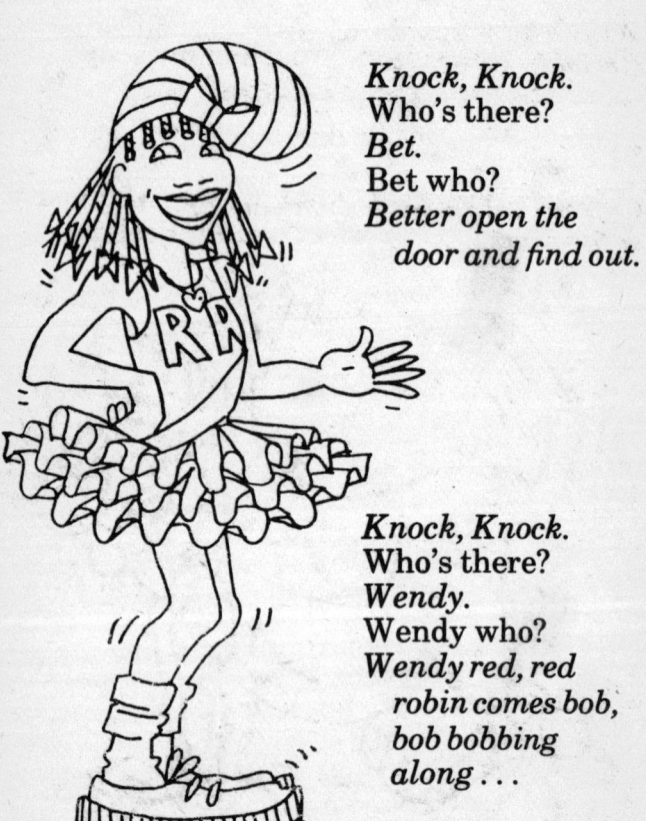

Knock, Knock.
Who's there?
Bet.
Bet who?
*Better open the
 door and find out.*

Knock, Knock.
Who's there?
Wendy.
Wendy who?
*Wendy red, red
 robin comes bob,
 bob bobbing
 along . . .*

Where do policemen look for clues?
Leeds.

Where do you look for eggs?
Egham.

'Waiter there's a cockroach in my soup!'
'Yes Sir, the fly is on holiday.'

'Doctor! Doctor! I think I'm a dog! But apart from that I'm in perfect health. Feel my nose.'

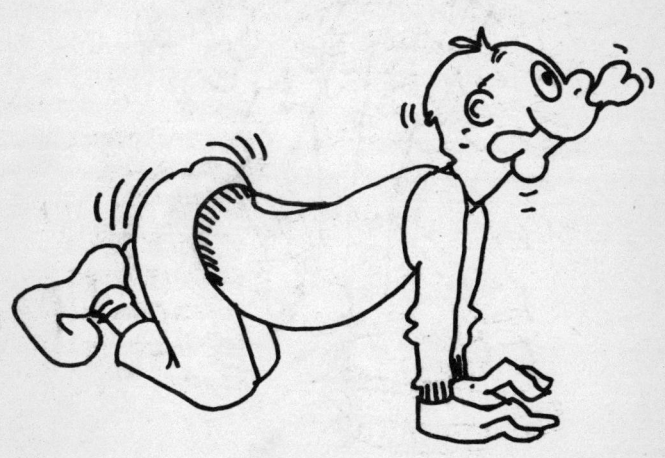

JUDGE: *You are a football hooligan . . . I find you guilty!*

HOOLIGAN: On what grounds, Your Honour?

JUDGE: *Well Chelsea, Wembley, Stamford Bridge . . .*

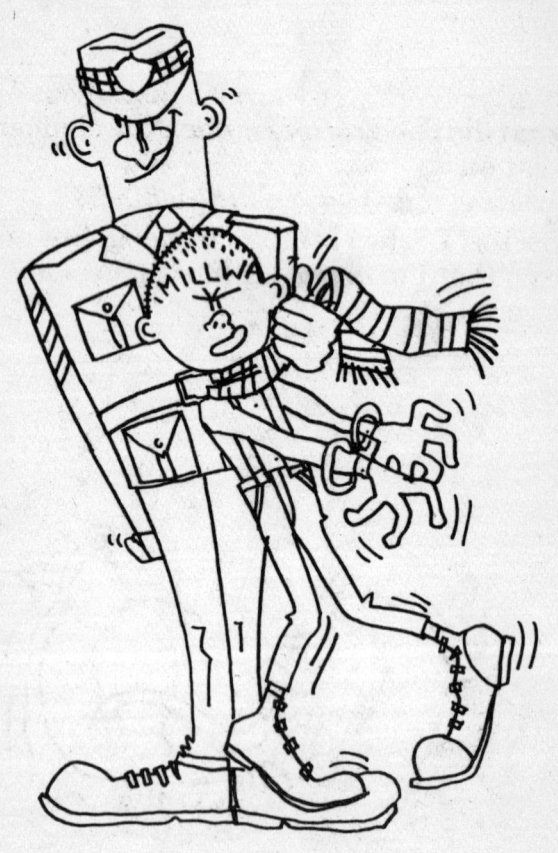

Where do clowns live?
Piccadilly Circus.

Where do you go to get a stopper for your
bottle?
Cork.

What did the grape say when the elephant
sat on it?
Nothing, it just gave a little whine.

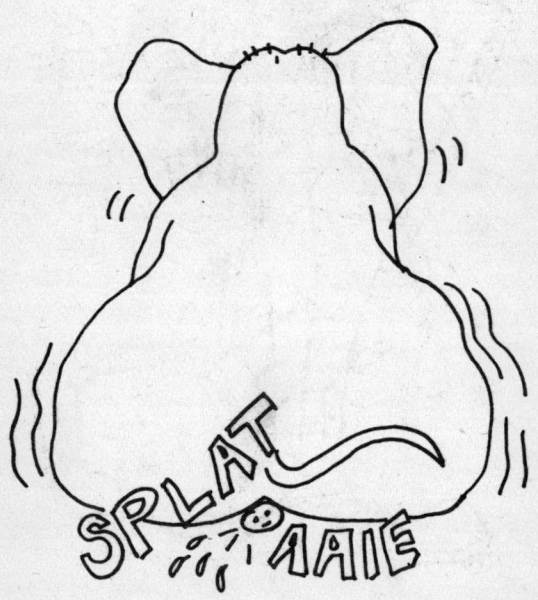

CUSTOMER: Waiter this fish is bad!
WAITER: *You naughty, naughty fish . . .*

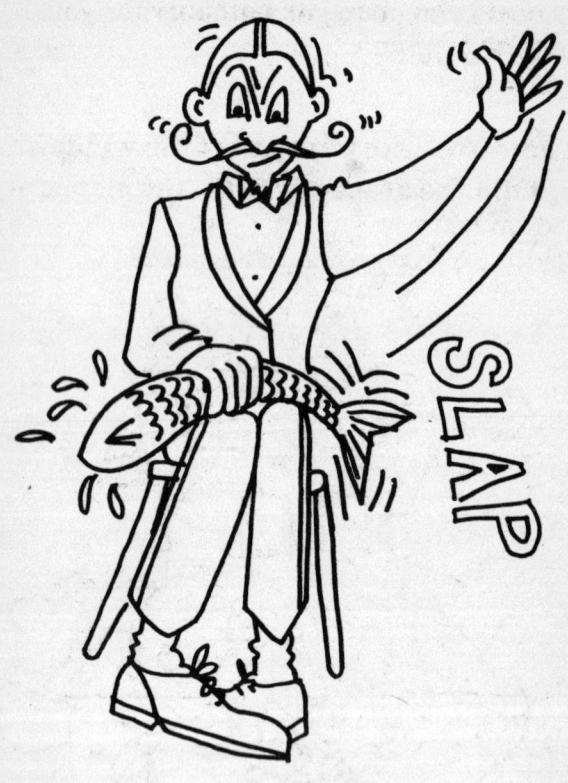

Where is the best place to go for Christmas
dinner?
Turkey.

What do frogs drink?
Croak a cola.

How does a bee keep its hair tidy?
With a honeycomb.

Why did Wallena jump out of the window?
To try out her new jump suit.

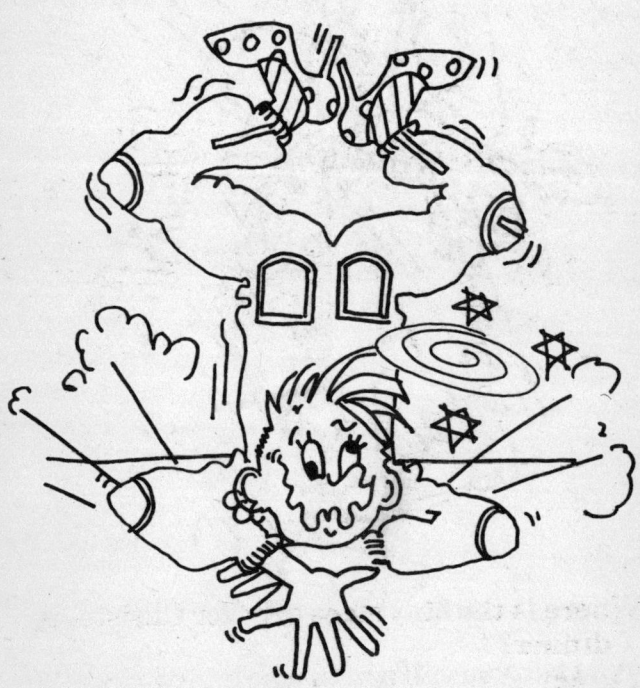

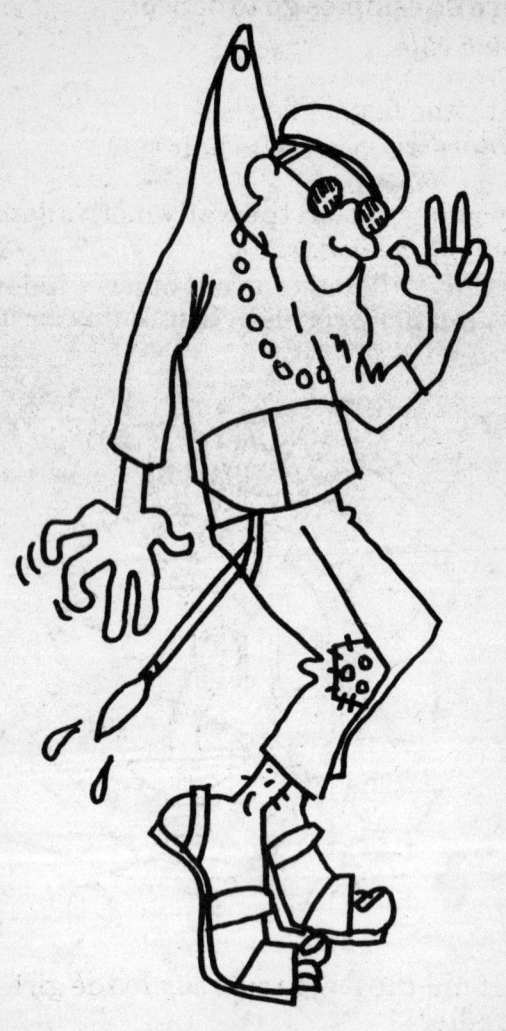

What do you call a man who hangs on walls?
Art.

Where do eskimos go to dance?
A snow ball.

What's the fastest fish?
A motorpike.

Did you hear about the wally morris dancer?
He fell off the bonnet.

What did little corn say to mummy corn?
Where's popcorn?

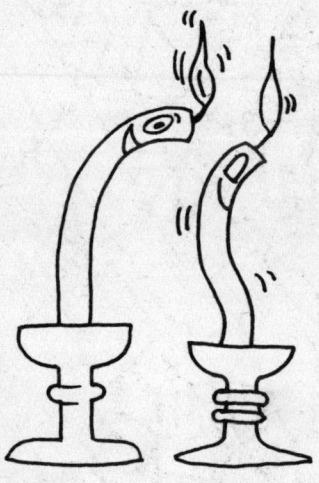

What did the boy candle say to the girl
  candle?
Do you want to go out with me tonight?

What do you call a cowboy who's always
  broke?
Skint Eastwood.

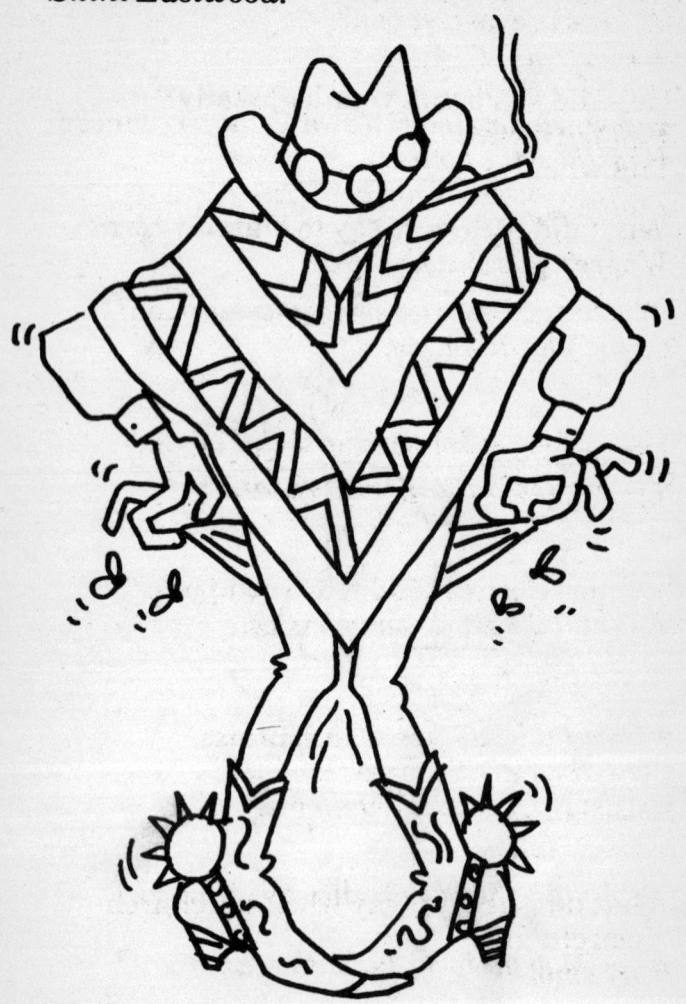

GET WELL SOON

2

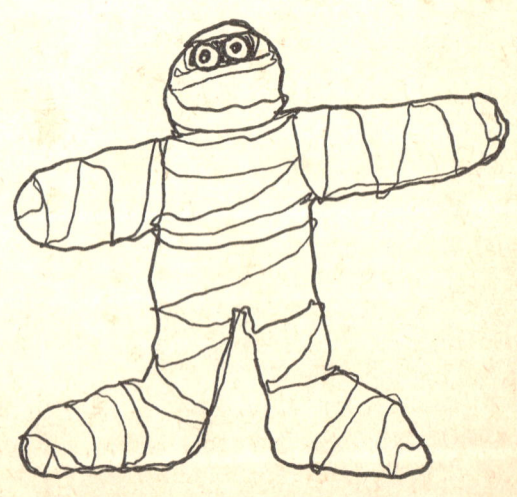

GEORGE EVANS

Get Well Soon

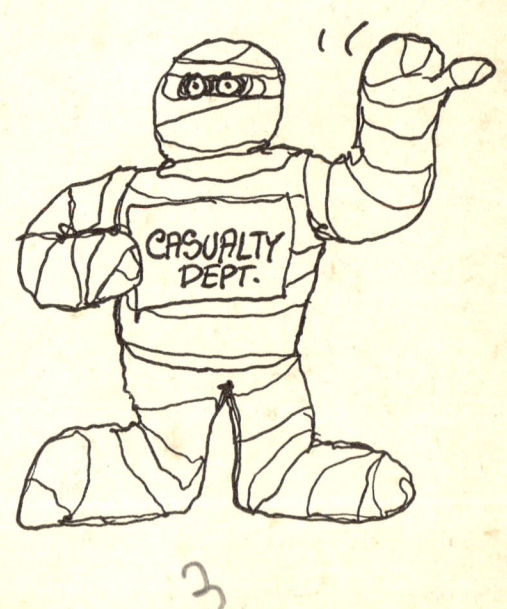

3

Futura
Macdonald & Co
London & Sydney

A Futura Book

First published in Great Britain in 1984
by Macdonald & Co (Publishers) Ltd
London & Sydney

ISBN 0 7088 2473 0

Typeset, printed and bound in Great Britain by
Hazell Watson & Viney Limited,
Member of the BPCC Group,
Aylesbury, Bucks

Futura Publications
A Division of
Macdonald & Co (Publishers) Ltd
Maxwell House
74 Worship Street
London EC2A 2EN
A BPCC plc Company

4

The General Practitioner

or,

The only person who enjoys poor health!

Doctor: Ah! Good morning, Miss Fullbody. I'd like you to remove all your clothes for an examination.
Miss F: Certainly, Doctor. Where shall I put them?
Doctor: On the floor, next to mine!

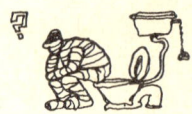

As the Doctor said when he handed the prescription to the marathon runner, 'Take one of these pills every half a mile!'

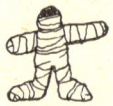

'Let me see, now,' said the Doctor, 'the pulse seems to be normal . . . blood pressure's all right . . . reflexes normal . . . heart normal . . . Good! Splendid, Mr Jones. *I'm* all right so let's have a look at *you*!'

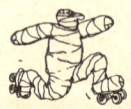

The Doctor handed the patient the prescription. 'Take this to your chemist and have it made up. It's the very latest tranquilliser – it doesn't relax you, it makes you enjoy feeling tense!'

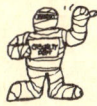

Doctor: So far so good, Mr Jones. Now I want you to fill that bottle over there, on the shelf.
Jones (surprised): You must be joking! From *here*?

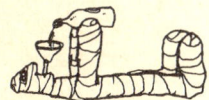

The receptionist at the Health Centre called out 'Next patient, please', and a dirty old tramp stood up and shuffled to the Doctor's office door. He knocked on the door, went inside and shuffled over to the Doctor's desk.

The Doctor finished filling in a form and looked up at the dishevelled heap standing humbly in front of him. His nose wrinkled up with distaste.

'You can't come in here,' he shouted. 'You're nothing but a dirty, stinking, filthy, nauseating, disgusting old tramp!'

The old tramp nodded. 'That's what the other Doctor told me,' he said, 'but I wanted a second opinion!'

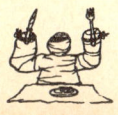

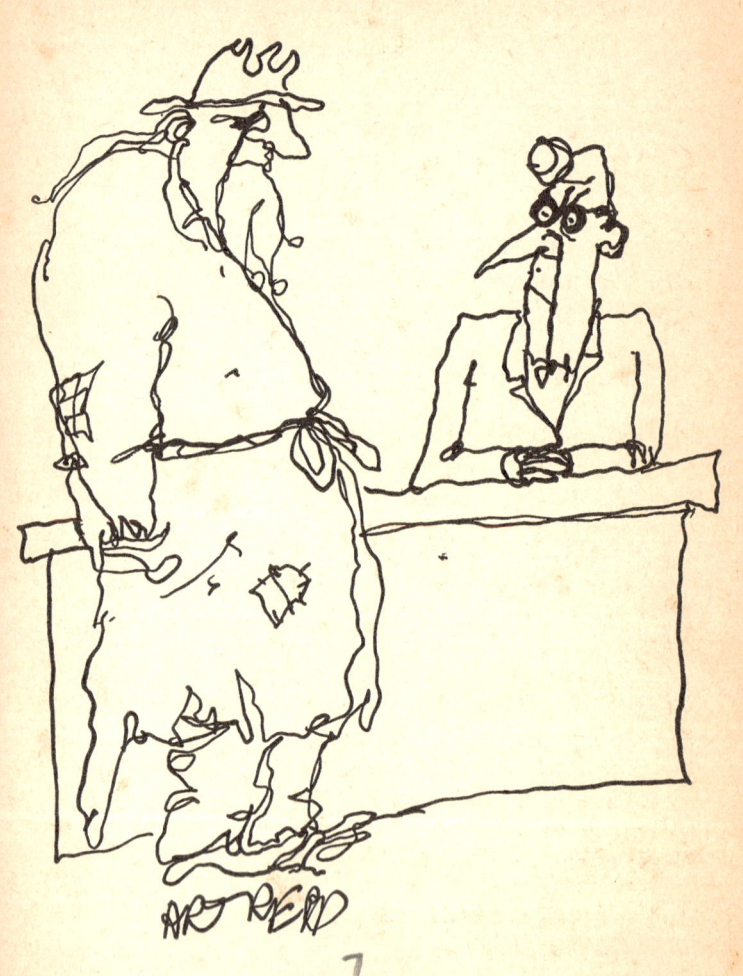

The Doctor's Surgery was packed. It was one of those 'there's a lot of it about' days. Suddenly, one of the patients, a very beautiful girl, gave a little cry, closed her eyes and slid peacefully from her chair and on to the floor in a dead faint.

The entire surgery came alive within seconds. 'Doctor,' they screamed, 'Doctor!'

The cry for help did not pass unnoticed. Immediately Dr Hudson, the one that all the lady patients asked for, stepped into the room and took in the situation with a single, expert glance.

'Right! Out of the way, everyone,' he ordered. 'Don't crowd her. Give the lady some room. I'm going to give her artificial recreation!'

There was a silence.

'Excuse me, Doctor,' murmured the local bank manager, 'but don't you mean artificial *resp*iration?'

The Doctor looked at him. '*You* give her what *you* want. *I'll* give her what *I* want!'

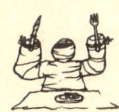

Or alternatively . . .

The handsome young Doctor was chatting up the beautiful Nurse Lovitt and trying to impress her.

'Well,' he said, 'this bathing beauty fainted, and they called for a Doctor! I was the only Doctor there!'

Nurse Lovitt stared at him with admiration in her eyes.

'What did you do then?' she breathed.

'Well,' he said, 'as soon as I saw her, I knew there was only one thing to do, so I did it!'

Nurse Lovitt leaned closer.

'I'll bet it saved her life,' she whispered huskily.

'It did, but I was only just in time. I had to give her artificial recreation.'

Nurse Lovitt stopped breathing and whispered huskily.

'But you mean artificial *respiration*! Artificial *recreation* is when you have fun.'

The handsome young Doctor faltered. 'Oh!' he said, 'you *saw* me.'

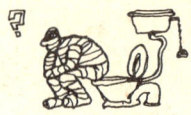

There are so many medical programmes on television these days: 'Your Life in Their Hands', 'Doctors' Dilemma', 'Kill or Cure?' One more and television's going on the National Health!

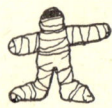

Doctor: Ah! Good morning, Mrs Allabright. What a beautiful morning, and to make it even better, I've got some *wonderful* news for you!
Allabright: But I'm not *Mrs* Allabright, Doctor, I'm *Miss* Allabright!
Doctor: Ah! . . . In that case, I've got *terrible* news for you!

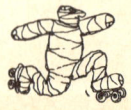

The two strong young men lifted the frail old chap on to the Doctor's couch and stood back anxiously as the Doctor bent over him and applied the smelling salts.

After what seemed an eternity, the old man moved and his eyes flickered open. For a second, he stared at the Doctor blankly, then recognition dawned.

'Oh, Doctor, Doctor,' he quavered, 'it was so sudden! All I can remember is the ambulance.'

The Doctor smiled gently. 'I'm not surprised, old friend. It was the ambulance that ran you over!'

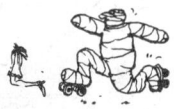

Then there was the Doctor who treated a patient for yellow jaundice for seven years before he realized he was Japanese!

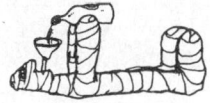

Doctor: Well, Mr Powell, you seem to be in very good condition to me. You can do up your shirt now, and if you wouldn't mind, I'd like you to walk over to that window, open it and poke out your tongue . . . that's it. Thank you very much!
Powell: Excuse me for asking, Doctor, but why did you want me to do *that*?
Doctor: Well, actually, I can't *stand* my neighbours!

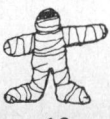

These days they have special vitamins for the younger child – B1, B2 and B-Quiet!

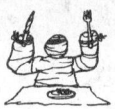

Patient: ... So it seems, Doctor, that I have a very serious memory problem. It's absolutely incredible, but I don't seem to be able to remember anything once I've said it!

Doctor: Mmmm ... interesting ... interesting. How long has this been going on?

Patient: How long has *what* been going on?

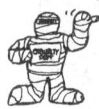

The beautiful blonde looked across the desk at the Doctor with a slight embarrassment showing on her face.

'Come on,' he encouraged her, 'I'm your Doctor. You can tell *me* what's wrong.'

'Well,' she said, with a self-conscious glance downwards at her admirable bosom, 'it's just that every time I get a cold, it always goes to my ... er ... my chest.'

'Never mind,' he smiled comfortingly. 'It just shows that it's got its priorities right!'

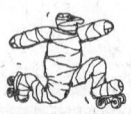

Patient: Oh, Doctor, Doctor, I had to see you! You've got to help me, Doctor! You've got to! I'm relying on you, Doctor! Please don't fail me, you're my only hope! Doctor... (*screams*) you've got to tell me, Doctor... why won't people speak to me? *Why won't they speak to me?*
Doctor: Next, please!

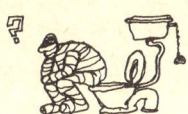

The old couple sat apologetically in front of the Doctor's desk, and hesitated. 'Er,' they said.

The Doctor smiled. 'Now for goodness' sake, Mr and Mrs Staples, you must tell me what's wrong! We've known each other for a long time now. You can tell *me*.'

The old couple looked at each other. Then Mr Staples spoke.

'Well, Doctor,' he said, 'it's like this... we've suddenly found that we're impotent.'

The Doctor shook his head. 'But, Mr Staples, you're eighty-five and your wife is eighty-three. It had to happen. When did you find out?'

He sniffed. 'Last night and again this morning!'

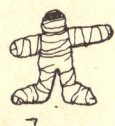

Patient: Just one thing, Doctor. When the bones knit together in my hands again, will I be able to play the piano?
Doctor: Of course you will!
Patient: That's funny! I couldn't play a note before!

Overheard in a Doctor's Surgery by a fly on the wall . . .
Patient: . . . and after the first, I'm slightly out of breath and a bit tired, then after the second my chest starts to ache and my heart starts to pound, and by the third – well, I honestly feel like fainting!
Doctor: But why don't you stop after the first?
Patient: I can't! I *live* on the third!

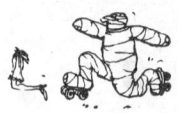

The Doctor finished examining old Mr Cooper.
   'Congratulations,' he said. 'At eighty-seven you're as good as ever! You're marvellous! I just can't believe it – eighty-seven years old and you're in the pink of condition! Wonderful!' He laughed, then added jokingly, 'How's your sex-life?'
   Mr Cooper smiled modestly. 'Almost every night,' he said. 'Thanks, Doctor.' And he left.
   A week or two later, the same Doctor finished examining old Mr Cooper's wife and pronounced her near perfect.
   'You're a marvellous couple,' he said, 'you and Mr Cooper! Eighty-seven, both of you, and still having a consistent love-life!'
   Mrs Cooper frowned. 'Consistent? You mean *non*-existent!'
   The Doctor blinked. 'But your husband told me you made love almost every night!'
   '*That's* right,' said Mrs Cooper. '*Almost* Monday night, *almost* Tuesday night, *almost* Wednesday night, *almost* . . .'

The Doctor looked up from studying the patient's records with a serious face.

'I think the best thing for you, old chap, is to give up drink immediately,' he said.

The patient winced.

'I don't deserve the best, Doctor,' he said. 'What's next best?'

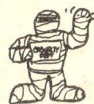

The pub was crowded, and the beautiful brunette was feeling the heat. Suddenly she gave a tiny, strangled sob and fainted. Luckily there was a young Doctor present, and in one, swift bound he was at her side, cradling her head in his arms. There was only one thing to do and he did it! He gave her the Kiss of Life.

Ten minutes later, he straightened up. 'Has it done the trick?' someone asked.

'Well, I don't know about *her*,' the Doctor said, 'but it did *me* the *power* of good!'

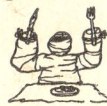

The next patient in to see the Doctor was a very pretty young girl, breathing heavily and looking upset.

'Oh, Doctor,' she breathed, 'please help me.'

'Calm down, Mrs Blythe, calm down,' he soothed. 'It sounds to me like a touch of asthma. Don't worry, it's not the end of the world.'

'It almost was,' she said. 'You see, I've just returned from my honeymoon . . . oh dear! I saved him just in time.'

'Saved who?' asked the baffled Doctor.

'My husband,' she sobbed. 'On our first night. It was all because of my asthma. He was going to jump off the balcony because he thought I was hissing him!'

14

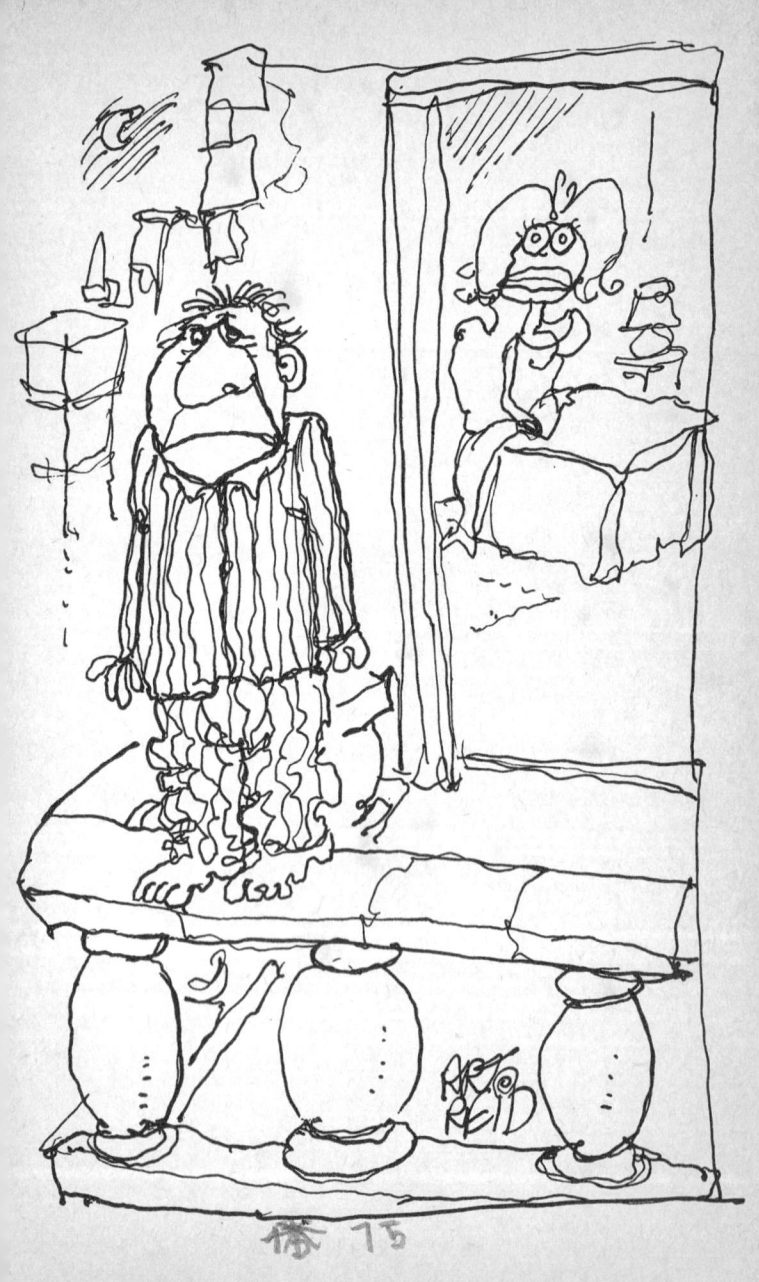

Then there was the rampant Old Maid who went to see the handsome Doctor.

Without waiting for him to ask her the problem, she immediately stripped off and said, 'Well, don't just stand there – examine me!'

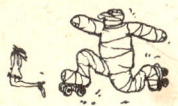

Doctor: Ah! Good morning, Miss Feltbody. And what's wrong with you this lovely morning?
Miss F: I've got laryngitis, Doctor.
Doctor: Then why aren't you whispering?
Miss F: It isn't a secret!

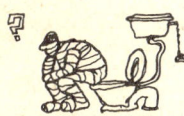

Medical Science has invented a new diet for ardent slimmers and weight watchers. You can eat anything you like, but don't swallow it!

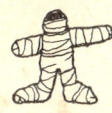

Patient: I seem to have lost all my energy, Doctor. I'm so listless I can't be bothered to do anything, only sit around!
Doctor: Mmmm . . .
Patient: Could it be something to do with my blood, Doctor?
Doctor: Mmmm . . .
Patient: Do you think another blood test would be any good?
Doctor: Normally, yes, but you've already had so many you're anaemic!

Then there was the shy but very beautiful young blonde. When the Doctor asked her to take off her clothes, she thought twice and then said, 'We-ell . . . all right, but only if you take me out first!'

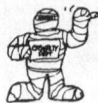

Doctor (gravely): I'm so sorry to call you in to see me, Pendleton, but I thought you ought to know that I'm very much afraid that your wife's mind has gone!
Mr P: Well, I must say I'm not surprised, Doctor. She's given me a piece of it every day for the last twenty years!

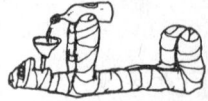

The Doctor was sitting at his desk just after his surgery had finished when a small boy and girl walked in. They couldn't have been more than six years old.

The Doctor smiled gently at them.

'I'm sorry, children,' he said, 'my surgery has finished. However, as you're here I suppose I can spare you a minute. What seems to be the problem?'

The little girl stepped forward.

'Doctor,' she said, 'Justin is six and I am five-and-three-quarters. Can we have children at our age?'

The Doctor smiled again.

'No,' he said, 'you can't!'

She turned to Justin.

'You see?' she said, 'I told you not to worry!'

The Doctor looked up.

'Well, Mr Cornball, and what seems to be the matter with you?'

The patient blinked painfully. He was obviously suffering.

'Well, Doctor,' he muttered, 'work over a lathe in a factory, don't I, and I've got some metal in my eye.'

The Doctor smiled. 'Don't worry, Mr Cornball, I've got the very latest in Japanese medical equipment that will do the job quite painlessly. It's called a magnet! Hold still, please.'

The Doctor held the magnet in front of the man's eye, and immediately twelve pieces of metal emerged from the eye and attached themselves to the magnet.

'There you are, Mr Cornball,' he said, 'I don't think you'll have any further trouble now.'

The man blinked. The Doctor was right. There was no pain.

'Doctor,' he said, 'I can't thank you enough.'

And as he walked to the door, the soles of his shoes fell off . . .

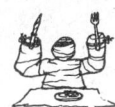

Doctor: I've made all the necessary tests, Miss Brestbury, and there really is no doubt at all. You are pregnant!

Miss B: But I don't see how it could possibly have happened, Doctor!

Doctor: Oh, it's easy enough, Miss Brestbury . . .

Miss B: But I don't think you quite understand, Doctor. You see, I belong to a new Nudist Order, and we are not allowed to make love as others do it. We only make love with our eyes.

Doctor: It's still easy, Miss Brestbury. Someone in your new Nudist Order is cock-eyed!

Doctor: How many children did you say you had, Mrs Pubes?

Mrs P: Twelve, Doctor, and I don't want no more! You got to give me something to protect me, Doctor.

Doctor (writing): I will, Mrs Pubes, right away! Take this prescription to the nearest chemist and have it made up. It's quite harmless. It's aspirin.

Mrs P: Thank you, Doctor. When do I take it – before, during, or after?

Doctor: Instead of!

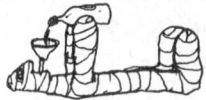

Doctor: Well, Miss Nightingown, I'm sorry to have to tell you this, but in my view you have acute appendicitis.

Miss N: Oh, Doctor, you *are* a darling, but I honestly came here to be *examined* – not flattered!

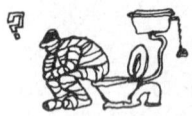

Doctor: Good morning, Mr Powell. Sit down. Now my advice to you is simple but urgent!

Mr P: And what's that, Doctor?

Doctor: Don't touch coffee, cigarettes, booze or Jackie Collins books!

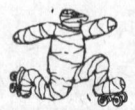

He's one of those progressive Doctors. He doesn't ask his male patients to stick out their tongues and say 'Ahhhh!', he just shows them a Bo Derek calendar!

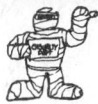

Mr Whitelaw: But, Doctor, what would you suggest was my best way to keep fit?
Doctor: In view of your busy schedule six days a week, I would suggest horse riding every Sunday.
Mr Whitelaw (startled): Horse riding! But is that all right for a sixty-three year old man?
Doctor: It is if you ride a sixty-three year old horse!

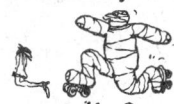

Mrs Lovitt, a very sad lady, went to see her Doctor.
'Oh, Doctor,' she cried bitterly, 'I can't sleep. I just can't sleep since my poor hubby went to meet his Maker. All night long, I just lie in my bed, tossing and turning. Them sedatives you give me don't do a thing, so I just tosses and turns, remembering all them idyllic moments we spent in bed together, making love.'
The Doctor was impressed.
'He must have been very accomplished,' he said.
'Oh, he was,' she cried, 'he was – specially on Sunday mornings!' Her eyes lit up at the thought.
'But why Sunday mornings?' asked the Doctor.
'Because on Sunday mornings,' she whispered huskily, 'the church bells used to chime, and we used to make love in time to them! Chime, chime, chime, they went, and chime, chime, chime *we* went . . . he was at his best making love to them bells . . . he'd have been here now if it hadn't been for that *bloody Fire Engine!*'

20

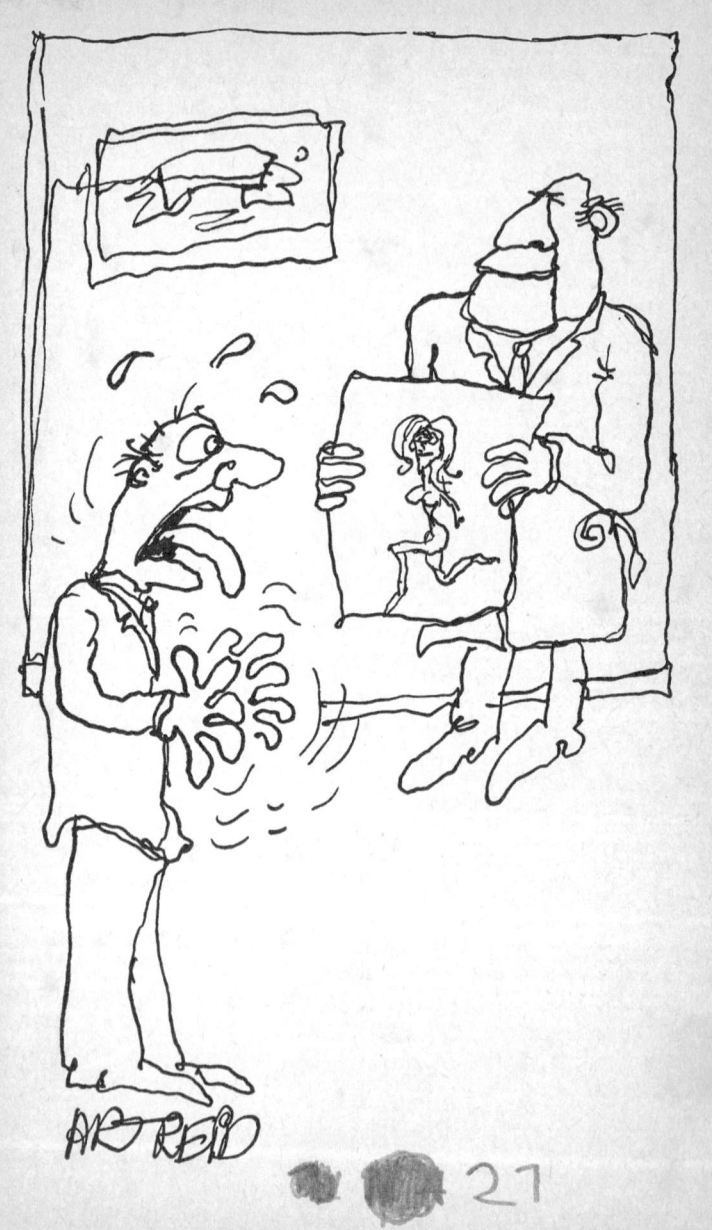

ARTREID

27

Then there was the drunk who went to see his Doctor with rheumatism of the hip. The reason for it? Spending too much time in pubs and putting wet change in his pocket!

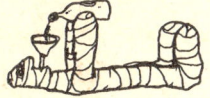

A man died of tuberculosis and was on his way to the cemetery in the hearse. Unfortunately it was involved in an accident and the casket was catapulted through the window of Boots the Chemist. As it passed the pharmacy counter the body sat up and said, 'Have you got anything to stop this coffin?'

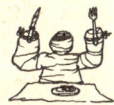

'Doctor, Doctor!'
'What seems to be the trouble?'
'I feel like I'm a pair of curtains.'
'Pull yourself together!'

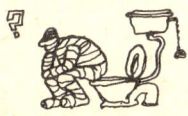

'Doctor, Doctor!'
'Yes, what's wrong?'
'I keep thinking I'm a billiard ball.'
'Go to the end of the queue!'

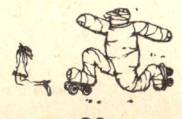

'Doctor, Doctor!'
'What seems to be wrong with you?'
'I keep thinking I'm a pack of cards.'
'Stop shuffling about. I'll deal with you in a minute!'

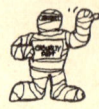

'Doctor, Doctor!'
'What's the problem?'
'I've got a cricket ball stuck in my throat.'
'Howzat?'
'Don't *you* start!'

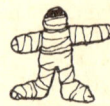

'Doctor, I feel like I'm a dog all the time.'
'How long have you had this problem?'
'Ever since I was a puppy.'
'Sit down over there for a moment.'
'Oh, but I'm not allowed on the furniture at home.'

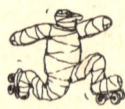

A man went to the doctor and reported back to his friend afterwards.

'The Doctor's given me some pills I have to take for the rest of my life, one a day.'

'What's wrong with that, doesn't sound so bad to me?'

'He's only given me five pills.'

Man goes to surgery. The doctor says to him, 'Hello, I haven't seen you for a long time.'

'I've been sick.'

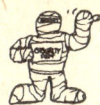

A man was told by his doctor to walk ten miles a day to alleviate a foot problem, and to report back to him in about four days' time. Time passed and eventually he rang up the doctor and told him it had got worse.

'Well, where are you now?' asked the doctor.

'Aberdeen.'

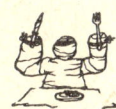

A man went to the Doctor's surgery to try and get a cure for his feet, which were smelly and had embarrassed him for some time.

The Doctor took a look at them and said, 'Well, put this foot powder on them and a new clean pair of socks each day and come back in five days' time.'

At the end of the week he came hobbling into the surgery. The Doctor took one look at him and asked him what the problem was. 'Well,' he said, 'now my shoes don't fit properly.'

The doctor took a closer look.

'That might be,' he said, 'because you've got five pairs of socks on!'

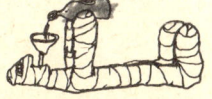

A man went to his Doctor and said, 'Hello, I wondered if you could give me anything for wind?'

The Doctor gave him a kite.

Nurses

or,

Just what the Doctor ordered —
but the chemist never had!

There was the gorgeous Nurse who made Dolly Parton look like a poor, under-nourished boy! She was so vain that every time she took a male patient's pulse she deducted twenty beats for her figure!

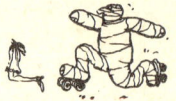

Nurse 1: Oooh, Sandra. Isn't Dr Williams terrific?
Nurse 2 (sighs): Mmmm . . . a dream . . . and he dresses so smartly.
Nurse 1: Yes — and so quickly, too!

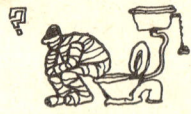

The ugly Nurse who became an operating-room Nurse because she looked better in a mask!

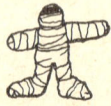

The religious Nurse who went around the male wards tucking the patients in for the night. Every time she tucked one in she sighed, *'Ah-Men!'*

The sexy Nurse who became a Nurse at an early urge!

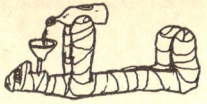

Nurse 1: Gillian, hear about Nurse Atkins? Well, I wouldn't say anything about Nurse Atkins unless it was good, would I – and, Gillian! *Is this good!*

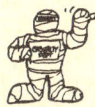

The patient who fell in love with Nurse Goodbody in Ward C.6. He plied her with champagne, flowers, chocolates and a fur coat.

They all worked!

Nurse 1: You know when I was at St Helier's Hospital, I was voted the Nurse most likely to.
Nurse 2: Likely to what?
Nurse 1: I don't know! I became pregnant before I could find out!

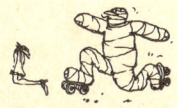

The sexy Nurse had to report to the Hospital Registrar for being late on duty.

He had her on the carpet, but she didn't seem to mind . . .

The Nurses of a well-known Hospital got together and wrote the following tribute to a very dedicated Doctor on the staff...

> 'Dr Newman is a handsome man
> Who has a lot of fun,
> He samples every pretty Nurse
> And never "Mrs" one.'

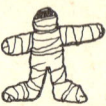

Sister: I really don't know, Nurse Bluett! Doctors! Doctors! Doctors! Is that all you think about?
Nurse B: You mean there's something *else*?

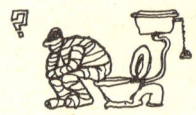

Nurse 1: Here, Sandra...
Nurse 2: What?
Nurse 1: Wonder why they call Nurse Atkins 'Appendix'?
Nurse 2: S'easy, isn't it? Take her out once, and that's enough!

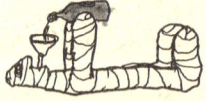

Then there was the inexperienced Nurse who fainted when the one-legged man asked her if she would hold his crutch for a minute.

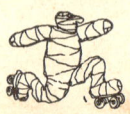

Gwyneth, a Nurse who was not all that well-blessed with looks and sex appeal was talking to her friend Brenda, also a Nurse in the same ward but who was just the opposite!

Brenda was the kind of a girl who kept going where Bo Derek left off!

'Guess what, Bren,' said Gwyneth, giggling, 'I've just bathed Mr Russell in Bed Twelve, and d'you know, he's got a word tattooed on his . . . well . . . you know – his Little Willie!'

Brenda laughed. 'Oh come on, pull the other leg – it chimes!'

'No, really,' giggled Gwyneth. 'Funny word, too! It's "Con" – C.O.N. – Con. Could be short for Connie, I s'pose – a girl-friend!'

Brenda still laughed.

'All right then,' said Gwyneth, 'if you don't believe me, *you* bath him tomorrow and see for yourself!'

When tomorrow came, Gwyneth and Brenda met again.

'Well?' said Gwyneth. 'Was I right or was I wrong?'

'You were right *and* wrong,' replied Brenda, with a big smile. 'You were right about there *being* a word, but you were wrong about the word – it wasn't *CON* – it was *CAERNARVON!*'

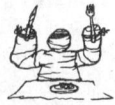

Wayward young Doctor: Oh, Nurse Proudpurse – just wondered if you . . . had anything on tonight.
Experienced Nurse P: Yes – and I'm going to keep it on!

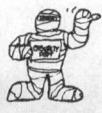

Nurse 1: Here, Sandra, is it true?

Nurse 2: Is what true?

Nurse 1: That Dr Holmes proposed to you.

Nurse 2: Oh, that! Yes!

Nurse 1: Well come on! What happened?

Nurse 2: I turned him down – *that's* what happened! I told him I wasn't that kind of a girl!

Nurse 1: But he only wanted to marry you!

Nurse 2: That's all you know! He said he wanted to have a practice in Brighton!

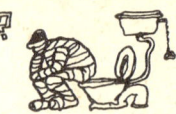

Nurse P: Hi, Sandra. Just on my way to see the Sister.

Sandra: Anything important?

Nurse P: Mr Hopkins in Bed Twelve didn't eat his breakfast this morning.

Sandra: Shame! Off his food, is he?

Nurse P: No. Dead!

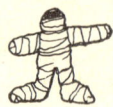

Or alternatively . . .

Nurse P: Hi, Sandra. Just on my way to see the Sister.

Sandra: Anything important?

Nurse P: Mr Salford in Bed Three didn't eat his breakfast this morning.

Sandra: Shame! Off his food, is he?

Nurse P (giggles): No, stupid! We never gave him any!

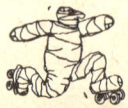

Then there was the flirty Nurse in the X-Ray Department — all her boy-friends saw through *her*!

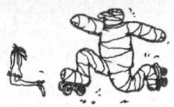

The Doctor and the beautiful Nurse looked at Mr Sodbury's chart.

'He's had a rough time, Nurse,' said the Doctor. 'We've got to do all we can to pull him through. Give him anything he wants.'

'I'll resign first,' she said.

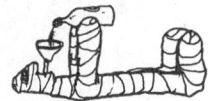

Sue: Hello, Lil. You're in a hurry!
Lil: Yes. I'm off to get some medicine to flush out alcohol from Mr Dexter's kidneys.
Sue: Has he got much alcohol *in* them?
Lil: I'll say! They're permanently stoned!

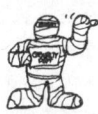

The Nurse who was always found in bed with a Doctor. No, she wasn't ill — she suffered from Virus Sex!

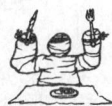

The patient was talking to two senior Nurses: '. . . Really,' he said, 'you don't look like sisters.'

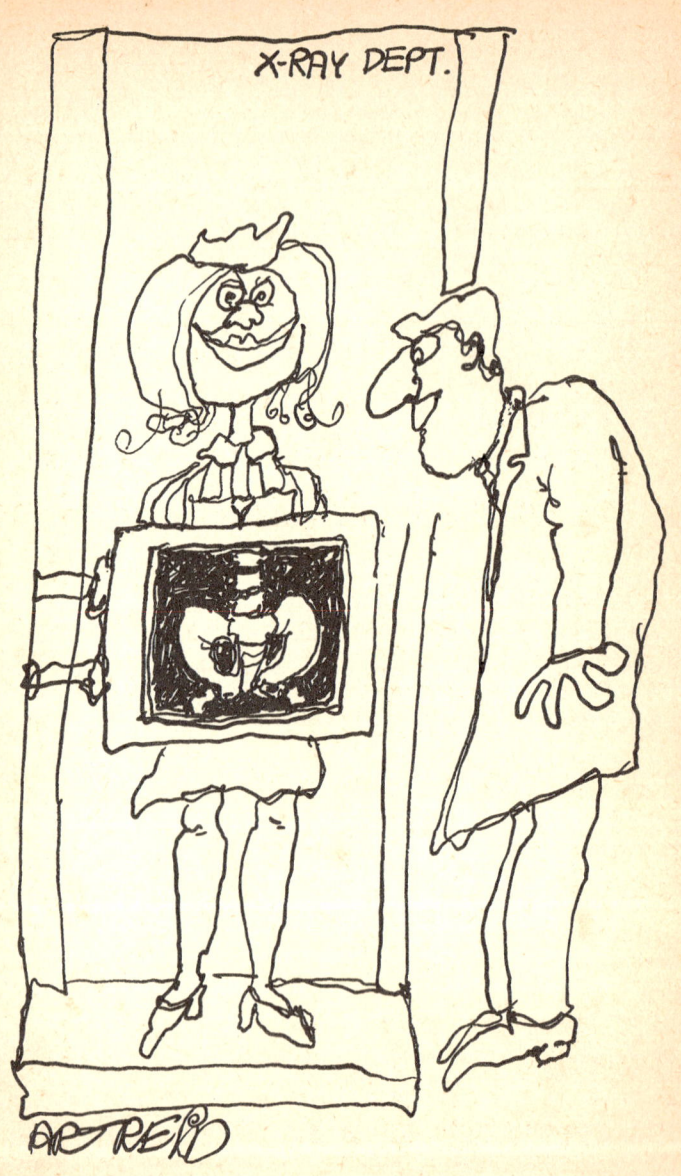

Doctorial Definitions

or,

Medical Meanings

Doctor: Someone with inside information.

*

Private Doctor: Someone who gives you an X-Ray to see how much you've got in your wallet.

*

Lady Doctor: Someone who intends to paint a patient's throat – when she can decide on the right colour!

*

Hospital: Where run-down people wind up.

*

Where the Nurses have all the curves and the Doctors have all the angles.

*

A place where you can lie around with time on your hands until six o'clock in the morning.

*

32

A place where they wake you up to give you a sleeping pill!

*

Anatomy: Something everybody has but it always looks better on a woman.

*

'The Lancet': (*Medical Journal*) The Eyes, Ears, Nose and Throat of the World.

*

Operation: Something that takes an hour or so to perform and a lifetime to describe.

*

Self-Service Operation: Where they open you up and help themselves.

*

Efficient Nurse: Makes the bed without disturbing the patient.

*

More Efficient Nurse: Makes the patient without disturbing the bed.

*

Priorities Nurse: Makes the patient first and the bed afterwards.

*

Private Medicine: Thar's Gold in them thar Ills!

*

Maternity Ward: A Bawlroom.

33

A Baby:	A hale fellow, well wet!

*

Paradox:	Two Doctors.

*

Conceited Ophthalmic Surgeon:	An 'I' Specialist.

*

Wisdom Tooth X-Ray:	Preview of a forthcoming extraction.

*

Psychiatrist:	The last person you talk to before you start talking to yourself.

*

A hypochondriac:	A man who likes to have his ache and treat it!

*

Someone who won't talk to you on the 'phone if you have a cold!

*

Someone who can't leave *being* well enough alone!

*

A person, who, on smelling flowers, looks around for the funeral!

*

A Sick Kleptomaniac:	Someone who takes things lying down!

Private Treatment

or,

A stitch in time costs money

It's wonderful to be a Private Doctor. In what other profession can you tell a beautiful woman to take off all her clothes and then send her husband a bill for it?

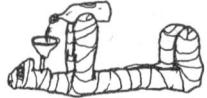

The millionaire lay in his private bed, in his private room, watching his private television set and happily working out how much he owed the private hospital after his operation.

He reckoned he owed them one thousand pounds for the room, five hundred pounds for the nursing, seven hundred and fifty pounds for the surgeon, two hundred and fifty pounds for the anaesthetist, and another two hundred pounds for his food, drink and morning papers.

Why was he so happy? Well he knew that with all that money to lose, they wouldn't *dare* let him die!

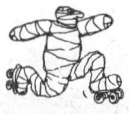

Surgeon 1 (after examination): Well, Mr Edwards, it doesn't look too good for him, does it?

Surgeon 2: No, it doesn't, Mr Corbett. I trust you'll go along with my decision?

Surgeon 1: Absolutely, Mr Edwards, all the way.

Surgeon 2: Good! In that case we'll remove the *whole* of his wallet!

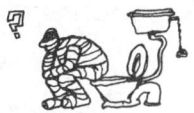

The Private Doctor who was private in every sense of the word. He was paid a hundred pounds a time for vaccinating strippers where it didn't show!

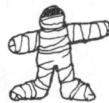

The patient was lying in bed in his room when he heard a polite knock on his door.

'Come in,' he called.

The door opened and a very attractive Nurse entered his room.

'Good morning, Mr Evans,' she smiled. 'Would you mind removing your pyjamas, please?'

Mr Evans did as he was told, and the Nurse then proceeded to put him through the most thorough examination he had ever had!

Finally she finished and told him that he could now don his pyjamas once again. Blushing, he did so as she smiled at him again and went to the door.

It was then that Mr Evans spoke.

'Oh Nurse . . .' he called.

She stopped and turned. 'Yes, Mr Evans?'

'Nothing much,' said Mr Evans, 'I just wondered . . . why did you bother to knock?'

Patient (softly): Nurse . . .
Nurse: Yes, Mr Marshall?
Patient: Give us a kiss.
Nurse: No, Mr Marshall.
Patient: Come on, Nurse . . . be a sport . . . just a kiss . . . just one . . .
Nurse: No, Mr Marshall. It's against the Hospital Rules . . .
Patient: Only one . . . come on . . . a *little* one . . .
Nurse: Certainly not, Mr Marshall! I shouldn't *really* be in *bed* with you!

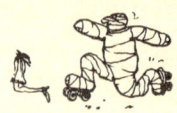

Doctor: Swab!
Nurse: Swab!
Doctor: Saw!
Nurse: Saw! Good Lord, Doctor, the patient's coming round!
Doctor: Circular saw!

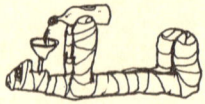

Then there was the Surgeon who always told his patients to eat a good meal before the operation! He hated working on an empty stomach!

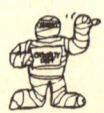

One Private Hospital wasn't doing so well and they had to make cuts!

Another Private Hospital wasn't doing too well, either. At one stage, they could only afford one stethoscope, and everyone had a party line!

Extract From the Diary of a Private Patient.
'Called to see my Doctor today for a "cheque-up". Funny how he always greets me the same way. "How d'you feel today", he asks me, stroking my pocket with the wallet in it . . .'

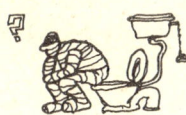

He's an M.D. until it comes to delivering babies. Then he's C.O.D.

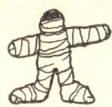

The Surgeon bent over the recumbent body of the very rich client lying on the operating table.

'Now don't worry, Mr Raygate. It's only a simple operation which won't take us very long. You won't feel a thing because we're going to give you a local anaesthetic.'

Raygate sat up on the table, his face purple with indignation.

'What?' he bellowed. 'You're giving me a *local* anaesthetic? Who the hell do you think you are! I don't *want* a local anaesthetic! I want the *best*! Give me the imported!'

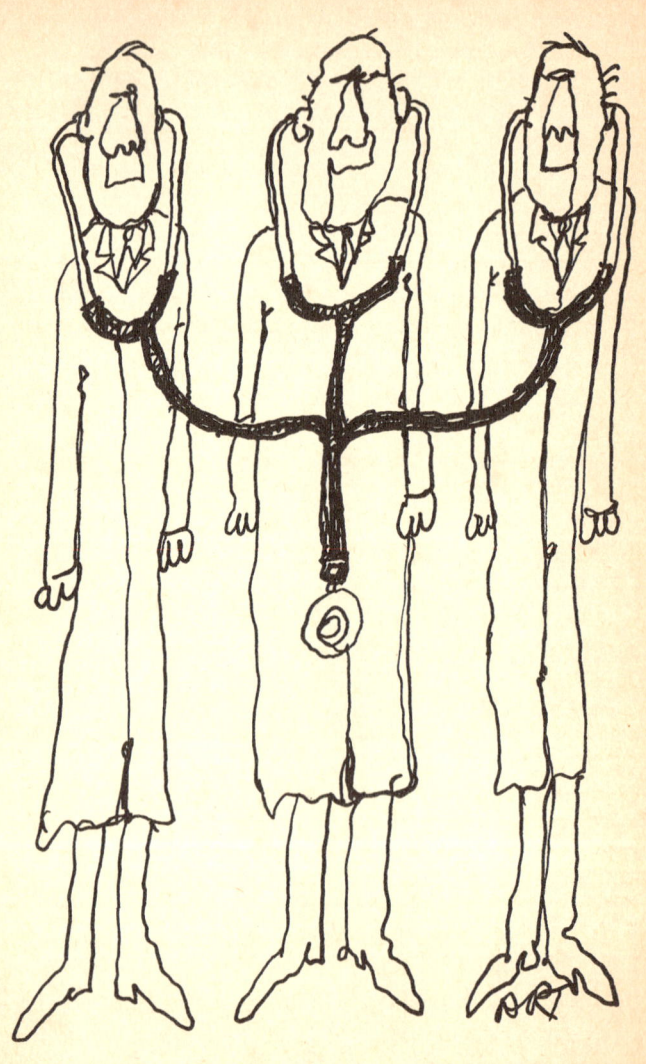

The millionaire was boasting to his visitor about the service in the Private Hospital.

'If you've got to be ill,' he said, 'this is the only way to live! It's wonderful here – just like a home from home ... food's marvellous ... wine is absolutely superb ...'

'How about the Nurses?' the visitor asked.

A glazed look obscured the millionaire's eyes.

'Out of this world,' he said, 'out ... of ... this ... world. I have one in the morning and another one in the evening.'

'What d'you do in the afternoons?' asked the visitor.

'What d'you *think* I do? I rest!'

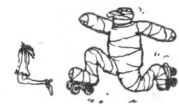

Not every Private Patient pays the bill on time. When they forget, they get a little note from the Hospital inscribed, 'Long Time, No Fee!'

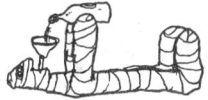

A certain Private Hospital caters exclusively for people who are not *quite* so rich! In their brochure, they advertise 'Every bedroom air-conditioned.'

Half-way through the afternoon, a Nurse comes in and squirts the room with an empty fly spray!

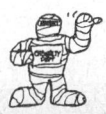

There was the money-conscious Private Doctor whose first words to a patient were, 'Open your mouth and stick out your cheque book!'

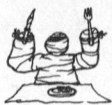

The Jewish patient who, on being told that his operation was to be featured in a well-known Television medical programme, exclaimed, 'My life! In their hands!'

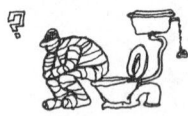

The millionaire who went into a Private Nursing Home to have the swelling removed from his wallet!

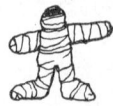

Doctor: Well, Mr Benny. You're getting all this throat trouble for one reason, and one reason only.
Benny: And what's that, Doctor?
Doctor: Your tonsils. I can take them out for you, but the operation will cost you £250!
Benny: (Thinks. Then . . .) Mmm . . . Tell you what, Doctor. If I give you a tenner will you loosen them a little?

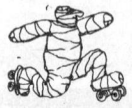

41

The Television Writer who left the Private Hospital and wrote a book about his experiences entitled, 'Your wallet in their hands!'

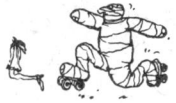

There was one vain woman patient who was so rich she went into a Nursing Home to have her gall stones taken out, and rhinestones put in!

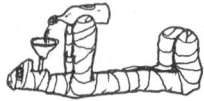

One patient was haggling over the fee for a physical examination. Finally, the exasperated Doctor said, 'All right, Mr Hudson. As a favour, I'll examine you in my own time for £50.'

'You're on,' said Hudson, 'but if you find it, we'll split it!'

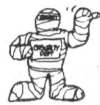

The Private Patient who had only been in hospital for a week before he found out the meaning of the medical term, 'Consultation'.

It was when his three Doctors got together to decide how to share out his money!

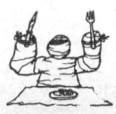

Patient: Hello Doctor. Good of you to see me so quickly. You see I've been suffering from the most terrible . . .

Doctor: Just a minute, just a minute, Mr Scruton! You do realize that I can't proceed any further with your case unless you pay me in advance.

Patient: Oh! No! Er . . . how much?

Doctor: Let's say . . . seven hundred and fifty pounds, shall we? Yes, let's!

Patient: Oh! All right then! Here's my cheque.

Doctor: Thank you, Mr Scruton. Well! That's *my* problem solved! What's yours?

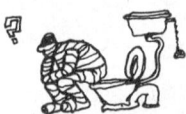

The rich man who woke up one morning and shouted 'Jeeves! I'm going to have a heart attack! Go and buy me a hospital!'

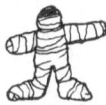

It was a small Private Nursing Home which advertised 'Semi-Private Accommodation' – two to a bed!

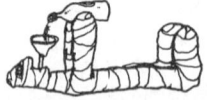

There was the Private Doctor who was ill but wouldn't treat himself because he was too expensive!

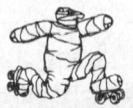

The Private Surgeon, Jewish by birth, Isaac Cohen by name, and skint by circumstances, sat in his office in despair. Everything had gone wrong, and now he was on the verge of bankruptcy.

Then the door opened and a wealthy-looking man came in.

'Mr Cohen?'

'I have that honour, yes.'

'Mr Cohen, I represent Mrs Gloria Woolmark!'

Mr Cohen's head swam. 'Mrs Gloria Woolmark – the richest woman in the western hemisphere! My life!' he thought.

'Oh, yes?' he asked politely.

'Mrs Woolmark,' the man continued, 'wants a face lift, and is willing to pay £20,000!'

Again, Mr Cohen's head swam. Twenty thousand pounds! It could be his saviour!

'Oh yes,' he said politely.

'Of course, it would have to be done by an expert surgeon – you *are* an expert Surgeon, I presume?'

'Oh, yes!'

'And you would undertake this operation?'

'Oh, *yes*!'

'It would have to be held a close secret, you understand.'

'May I be split asunder if I ever breathe a word about it,' muttered Mr Cohen, reverently.

'Good,' said the man. 'Then the job is yours! Oh!' he added quickly, 'there is just one, small snag.'

'Oh, yes?' asked Mr Cohen, hardly daring to breathe.

'The thing is,' said the man, 'are you Jewish?'

Mr Cohen thought carefully for a few seconds, then spread out his hands.

'Not necessarily,' he said . . .

The Irish Connection

or,

Hospital daze!

Did you hear about the Irishman on picket guard during the National Health strike? He stood outside the exit!

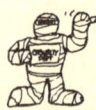

Mrs O'Brien: To be sure, Mrs Murphy, Fitzgerald's Maternity Home is a fine place for anyone wanting to have a child – if they are a woman, that is!
Mrs Murphy: And I wouldn't be disagreeing with you there. I'm told they've had some very famous births here in their time, too . . . really *big* people!
Mrs O'Brien: Ah, you're wrong there dear – only babies!

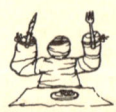

Doctor: Now, Mr O'Flynn, what seems to be the matter with you, today?
O'Flynn: I'm in terrible pain, sir. An Alsatian bit me on the finger.
Doctor: Which one?
O'Flynn: I don't know, sir. These Alsatians all look alike to me!

Then there was the Irishman who went into Hospital to have his head examined, but they couldn't find anything!

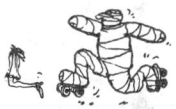

Mrs O'Brien: 'I hear that Shamus is going into hospital for a brain operation, Mrs Murphy. It must be very worrying for you.'
Mrs Murphy: 'Not at all, not at all, Mrs O'Brien. It's only a minor operation – they're putting one in!'

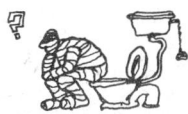

The Doctor finished examining Mr O'Brien's feet.

'Well, Mr O'Brien,' he said, 'there's nothing to worry about. All that's wrong with your feet is what we, in the medical profession, call Athlete's Foot! No, Mr O'Brien,' he said, raising his hand to stop Mr O'Brien's protests, 'I know you're never been an athlete! This is just an infection. Just sprinkle the powder on your feet, and very important, put on a fresh pair of socks every day! Next please!'

Mr O'Brien was back to see the Doctor within a week.

'You know you told me to put on a fresh pair of socks every day, sir,' he said.

'Yes,' said the Doctor.

'Well, I've done that, sir,' said O'Brien, 'but now I've got another problem – I can't get me shoes on!'

46

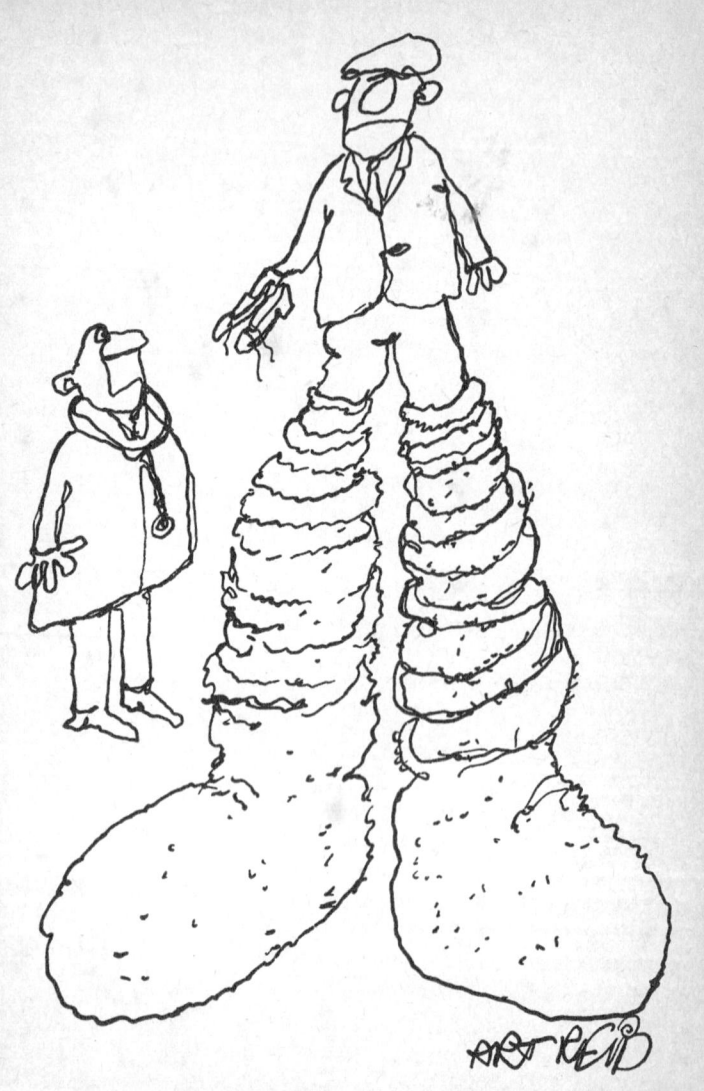

An Irish Male Nurse stayed up all night studying to pass his Blood Test!

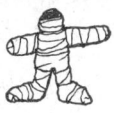

There was the Irish Surgeon who went around the hospital boasting that up to date he'd operated twenty-five times and only cut himself once!

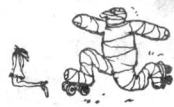

Doctor: I've received the report from the Gynaecologist, Mrs Murphy, and he's got exciting news for you. He says that you're going to have twins.
Mrs Murphy (angry): Sure and it's a demented lie! I've never been on a double date in me life!

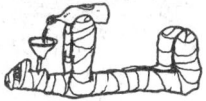

The Doctor leaned forward.

'If you really *want* to stop smoking, a good way is to find something else to take its place, Mr O'Rourke. Have you tried chewing gum?'

'Oh, yes, sir,' said Mr O'Rourke, 'but it was a failure all right. I couldn't get it to light!'

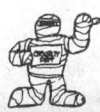

Mrs Murphy: And how's that son-in-law of yours, Mrs O'Brien?

Mrs O'Brien: Sure and he's studying to be a Plastic Surgeon.

Mrs Murphy: High and mighty! You'd think he'd want to be flesh and blood like all the others!

Doctor: You know, Shamus, I've never met such an incompetent, idiotic knucklehead before in my life! Sometimes I think your Nanny dropped you on your head when you were born!

Student: Oh no, she didn't, sir, we was too poor to be able to afford a Nanny – me Mammy had to do it!'

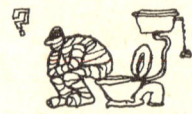

The Irishman who woke up one morning and found he had water on the knee, water on the elbow and water on the brain . . . so he got up and switched off the shower!

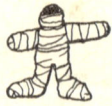

Mr O'Rourke: Doctor, I think I've got too much iron in me blood!

Doctor: What makes you think that?

Mr O'Rourke: I've got 'nails' on me finger-tips!

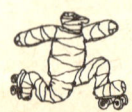

There was the Irish Plastic Surgeon who suddenly went out of business! He started to sign his work!

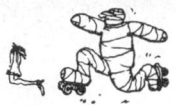

Pat: Faith, Mike me boy, is the truth true that I'm hearing that your fifth-born has just cut his first tooth?
Mike: It is and all, and wasn't I telling Esther he was too young to be playing with knives!

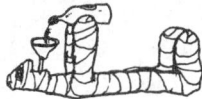

There was the Irish Surgeon who was talking about his earlier experiences to a friend of his. He said, 'And you know, I'll never forget my debut in the Operating Theatre in Belfast – and did dey boo!'

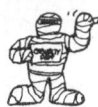

Surgeon 1: Mr O'Reilly, you *must* be more careful! This is the third Operating Table you've ruined this week and they're expensive! In future, please try to be more careful!
Surgeon 2: All right then! If you're so clever, p'raps you can tell me how!
Surgeon 1: Well – try not to cut so *deep*!

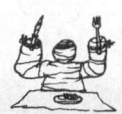

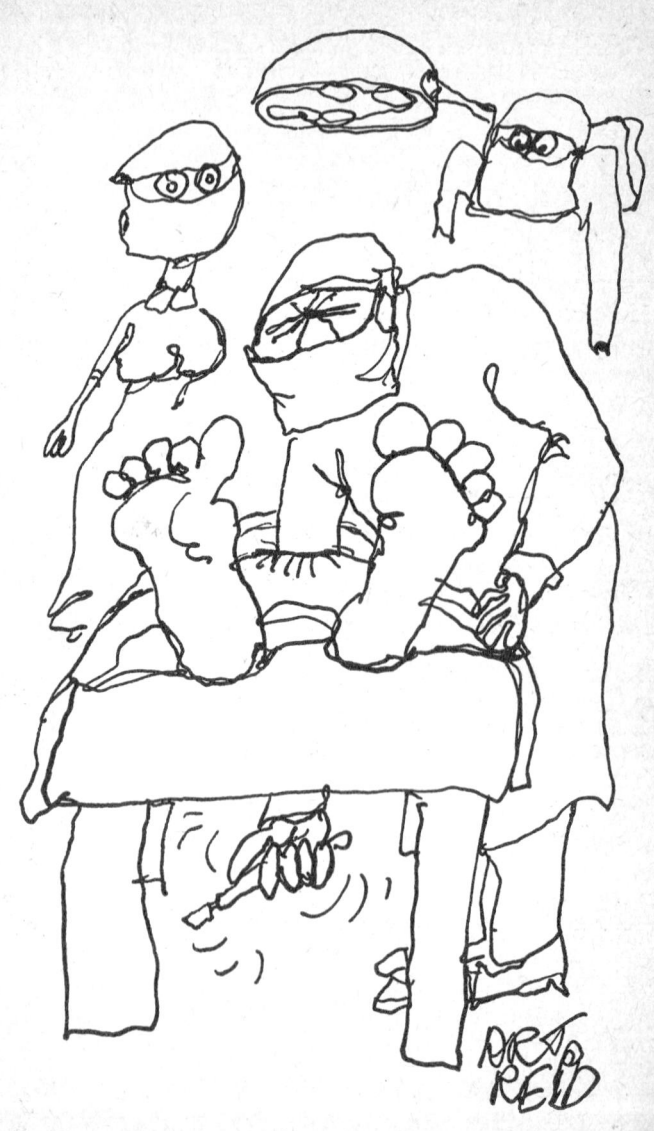

Then there was the young Irish couple who spent the first three weeks with their newly-born son poking a broom in his face. They wanted to get him used to kissing his grandfather!

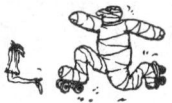

The Irish Medical Student who turned down the chance of becoming a Plastic Surgeon, in case he should melt when he went near a fire!

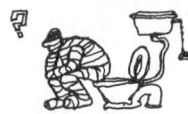

Then there was the Irish patient who shouted, 'Water! Water!' Straight away they knew he was delirious!

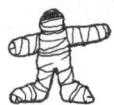

The Doctor examined Murphy's hands.

'Mmm,' he said, 'your hands *are* badly burned, Mr Murphy. How on earth did you do this?'

'Well, sir,' said Murphy, 'I was trying to drown the wife in a bath of acid, and I burned me hands pulling out the plug!'

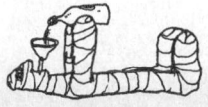

Bridget: Top of the mornin', Maureen. And what's this I hear about you havin' a baby?

Maureen: What you're hearin' is right, Bridget, sure enough, but it won't be until after Christmas.

Bridget: And why not Christmas? Sure, t'is a wonderful time for having children.

Maureen: Maybe so, Bridget, but they say deliveries are so slow over the holidays!

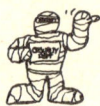

Mrs Kelly: Hello, Mrs O'Rourke! And how's the daughter's new baby?

Mrs O'Rourke: To tell you the truth, Mrs Kelly, we're all a bit disappointed with him! He only weighs three pounds seventeen ounces!

Mrs Kelly: Hardly worth bothering about, to be sure!

Mrs O'Rourke: It was on the tip of me mind to tell her to leave him in Hospital, and then I thought she might as well bring him home – it's better than nothing!

Doctor: Ah, Mr O'Mally. How's Mrs O'Mally and the new baby?

O'Mally: That's what I'm puzzled about, Doctor. The wife's gone raving mad! She's sent me around for a prescription for baby oil!

Doctor: But what's wrong in that?

O'Mally: Well, I've spent the last half-hour moving his arms and legs in all directions, but I can't get a squeak out of him!

Songs for Swinging Nurses

To: *Rupture Patients:*	'I'm Hernia Strolling Vagabond, So *Goodnight*, Pretty Maiden – *Goodnight!*'
	*
Indian Lady Doctors:	'The Sari With The Syringe on Top!'
	*
The Surgeon who removed a troublesome organ from a Jewish lady:	'My Yiddish Yam-aha!'
	*
The father of twins:	'T'Ain't What You Do, It's The Way That You Do It!'
	*
The Surprised Father:	'Is You Is, Or Is You Ain't My Baby?'
	*
Nurses who date fast Doctors:	'From Here To Maternity!'
	*
Doctors who date fast Nurses:	'From Here To Paternity!'

*

Varicose vein patients:	'Deep Purple!'

*

Asthma sufferers:	'Hay There!'

*

Anaesthetists:	'Happy "Daze" Are Here Again!'

*

New-born babies:	'Rock-a-bye Baby on the tree top, If the bough breaks it's a heck of a drop!'

*

All patients who have to give a sample:	'You ferment for me.'

*

Patients for dental treatment:	'I Saw You Last Night and got that Gold Filling.'

*

Visiting undertakers:	'To Each His Urn.'

*

All babies:	'There'll Be Some Changes Made.'

*

Heart transplants:	'My Heart Belongs To Daddy.'

*

Heart donors:	'I Left My Heart in San Francisco.'

'Onwards, "Christian" Soldiers!'

*

Nurses who shave patients for operations:

'Nobody Knows the Stubble I've Seen!'

*

'Ain't Misbehavin', Just Shavin' My Love, For You.'

*

'Little Things Mean A Lot!'

*

'I Got Plenty of Nuthin'.'

*

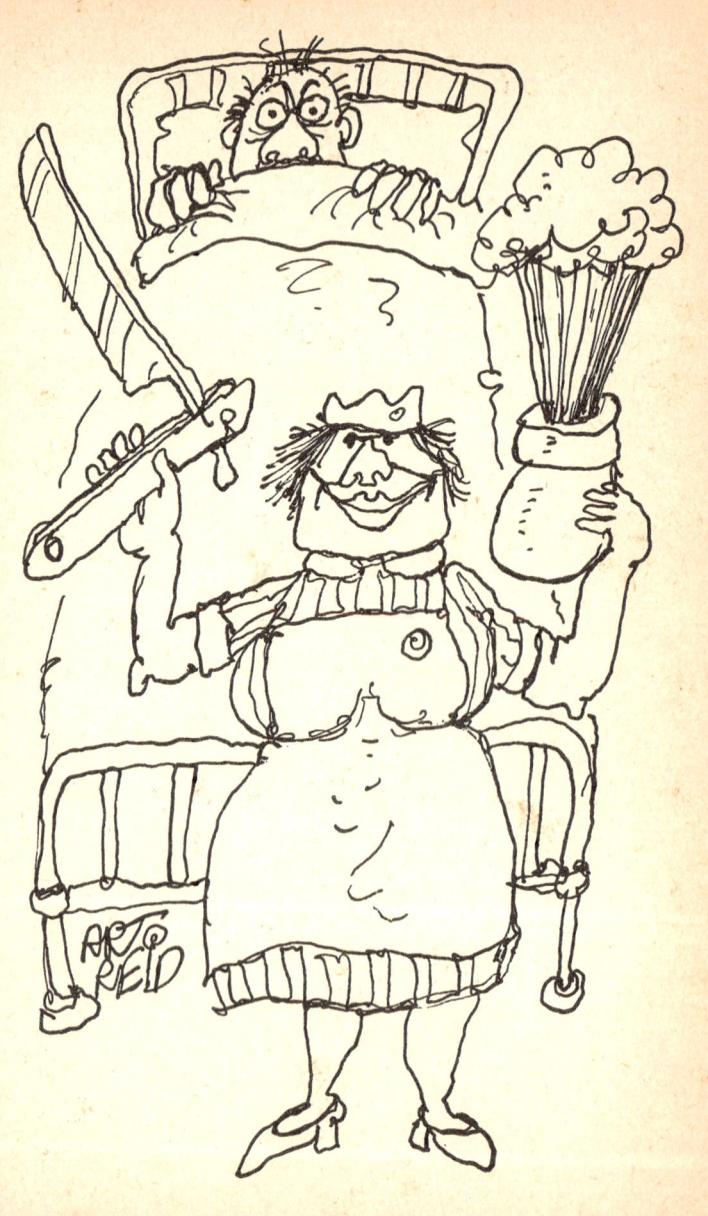

Out-Patients

or,

Patients are a virtue!

The man who went to Out-Patients because he'd swallowed a thermometer. He thought he was dying by degrees!

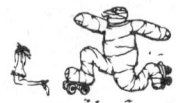

'Mr Collins!' called the Nurse, and the man with the nose looking like a piece of gorgonzola reeled off his chair and staggered into the Doctor's office, where he stood swaying in front of him.

'You wanted to see me?' said the Doctor.

'Yes,' slurred Mr Collins, breathing alcohol fumes all over him. 'I wondered if you'd be good enough to give me the address of Alcoholics Anonymous.'

'Of course,' smiled the Doctor. 'You want to join?'

'I've already joined,' hiccoughed Mr Collins, 'I want to *resign*!'

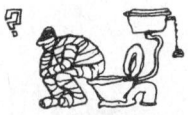

Mrs Smith: 'Aving another one, dear?

Mrs Hardly: No – lorst the button off-of me coat, that's all!

The Nurse standing by the weighing machine called out, 'Mrs Golightly!' and a very large lady took off her shoes and stood on the weighing platform as the Nurse weighed her.

'What do I weigh?' whispered Mrs Golightly.

'Eleven stone eight pounds,' said the Nurse.

'I wonder if you'd do me a favour and put me down as nine stone six?' simpered Mrs Golightly.

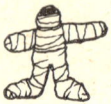

Mrs Hardly: Oh yes, dear, I'll always remember Tooting . . . there'll always be a part of me in Tooting . . .
Mrs Smith: Reely?
Mrs Hardly: Oh yes – I had me tonsils removed there!

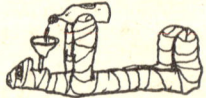

Mrs Smith: What *you* doing here, dear?
Mrs Hardly: Fell down stairs.
Mrs Smith: Missed a step, eh?
Mrs Hardly: No – hit every *one* of the ruddy perishers!

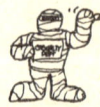

Mrs Smith: Can't understand it! I've been taking Vitamins A, B, C, D, E, F and G, and I *still* look like 'H!'

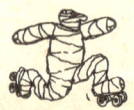

The pretty girl with the toilet seat ringing her shapely bottom stood in front of the grinning Doctor, her face red with embarrassment.

'I'm sorry,' apologised the Doctor. 'I really shouldn't laugh, but how on earth did you come to end up – if you'll pardon the expression – with this toilet seat stuck to you in the first place?'

'Well,' said the girl, 'I was at this party, and one or two of the fellows got a bit tiddley and thought it would be hysterical to paint the loo seat.'

'They didn't tell anyone.'

'No, there would have been no joke if they had,' she said. 'If you can call it a joke. Anyway, I was the unlucky one. I sat on the thing and it must have been very tacky when I did, because when I wanted to get up, I couldn't! The seat had dried! I'd locked the loo door, naturally, so they had to break down the door to get in, and no-one could shift it, so they unscrewed it, so here I am, seat and all!' She giggled. 'I don't suppose you've seen anything like this before!'

The Doctor grinned.

'Well actually I have, but this is the first time I've seen it framed!'

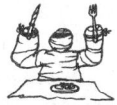

'Hello, Mrs Fulcrum, baby all right?'

'Oh yes, dear, thank you. He's almost six weeks, now.'

'Mmmm. Made up his mind what he's going to be when he grows up, then, has he?'

'Not quite, but we think he's going to be a politician.'

'Really? Why?'

'He wriggles out of everything we put him in!'

60

Rodney: Hello, Clive. Fancy seeing you here. What's wrong?

Clive: Nothing, Rodders, absolutely nothing!

Rodney: Fascinating! Absolutely fascinating! Then what are you doing in here in the jolly old Out-Patients?

Clive: I'm here with my friend Justin.

Rodney: Good Lord! Old Justers! What's wrong with the poor chap?

Clive: Something *ghastly*! He's swallowed a door-knob and it keeps turning in his stomach!

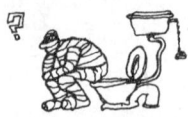

Woman (in panic): I say! Help! *Anybody!* I've just lost two children somewhere in Out-Patients! I wouldn't *mind*, but they're not mine!

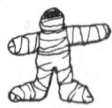

'Oh yes,' the woman said to her friend. 'I'm here to see the Specialist. No-one lower will do.'

'It must be important then,' said the friend.

'It is,' said the woman, 'it is! I've got trouble with my eyes. My Doctor says I've got a misplaced rectum . . .'

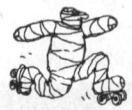

George: Hi, Frank. You look worried!

Frank: I ought to! I've just seen the Specialist and he says I need a complete overhaul!

George: What's wrong, exactly?

Frank: My kidneys don't know their onions ... my blood's an absolute clot ... any more water on the knee and I'll need a tap on my shin ... my armpits need protection ... my tongue is depressed, and my abdomen is rumbling so loudly my bowels are thinking of moving!

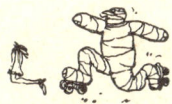

'Nigel! What are *you* doing here?'

'Waiting for Felicity. She's in with the Gynaecologist. She's having a baby.'

'Good for Felicity! I didn't know she had it in her!'

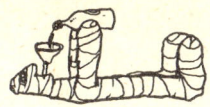

'And between you and me, Featherstone, the Specialist's a fool!'

'What makes you say that, old man?'

'Well, he told me to cut out drink and women.'

'So?'

'So I'm going to cut out drink! I can always drink when I'm old!'

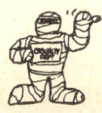

'My sister Lil was in this hospital . . .'

'Reely?'

'Yes . . . two days for observation.'

'Reely!'

'Yes. She said while she was in she never touched the food . . .'

'Bad, was it?'

'Dunno – they never give 'er any!'

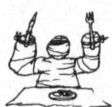

'. . . and I weigh eight stone eleven dressed, and nine stone three stripped.'

'Unusual. How's that?'

'Very heavy goose pimples!'

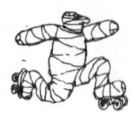

Food, Hospital Food!

or,

It must be jelly 'cos Jam don't shake like that!

The Hospital Kitchen Supervisor who wouldn't allow them to serve the patients breast of chicken unless it was in a bra!

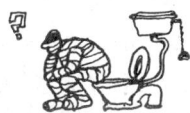

The coffee gave you grounds for anaesthetic!

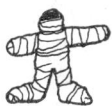

Sister: Mr Evans, we've had some complaints about our food.
Mr Evans: Really?
Sister: Yes. Now what did you think of dinner last night?
Mr Evans: Very tasty – in fact I can still taste it now!

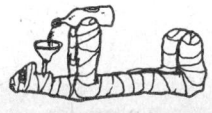

The Kitchen Supervisor who issued stomach pumps with every meal!

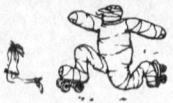

There's only one thing to say about Hospital Food – *'Burp!'*

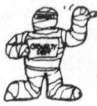

For dessert, they gave the patients what they called 'Two-handed Cheese!'
  You ate it with one hand and held your nose with the other!

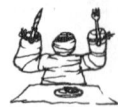

The main meal was what they called 'Scruples Stew'. They served it with reservations!

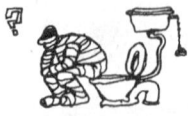

Even their breakfast cereal didn't go 'Snap, crackle and pop!'
  It just lay there and hiccupped!

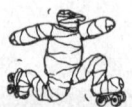

For dinner in the evenings, the Hospital boasted a seven-course meal – six beans on a piece of toast!

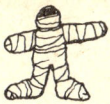

They'd heard of bad cooks before, but this was the first time the patients had had burned cole slaw!

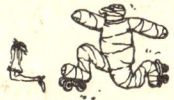

They were terribly slow in serving the food from the kitchen. One man put his tick by lamb, and when he got it, it was mutton!

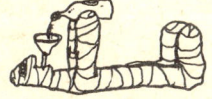

Operations

or,

May I cut in?

He was operated on so much he had a swing door put in!

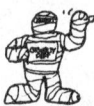

One Doctor specialized in appendix operations – he wanted to make some money on the side!

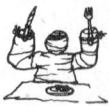

They say that the appendix is a useless organ. Perhaps so, but it's kept a lot of hospitals going!

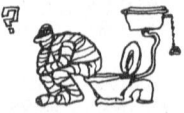

There was one man who needed so many stitches the Surgeon used a sewing machine!

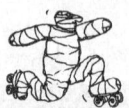

The patient awoke in a daze after his operation. Gradually the mists cleared a little, and he saw a hazy figure in white bending anxiously over him. He summoned up what he hoped was a smile.

'Was – was the operation a success, Doctor?' he croaked weakly.

'I'm frightfully sorry, Mr Prendagast,' said the figure apologetically. 'I'm not the Doctor – I'm St Peter!'

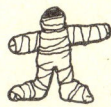

Professor Stitchley and his medical students were watching an operation.

Then the Professor asked the students, 'Can anyone tell me this? Which part of the human body is harder than steel?'

There was a silence.

'Come on, someone,' barked the Professor. 'Which part of the human body is harder than steel? Miss Loverjoy, you tell us!'

Miss Loverjoy's face went red, and she sniggered, 'Oh, *please* don't ask *me*, Professor!'

'All right,' rasped the Professor angrily. 'I'll tell you! The answer is nail tissue, and *you*, Miss Loverjoy, are the supreme optimist!'

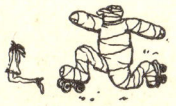

Why do Surgeons wear masks when they are performing operations? Because if anything should go wrong, nobody can identify them!

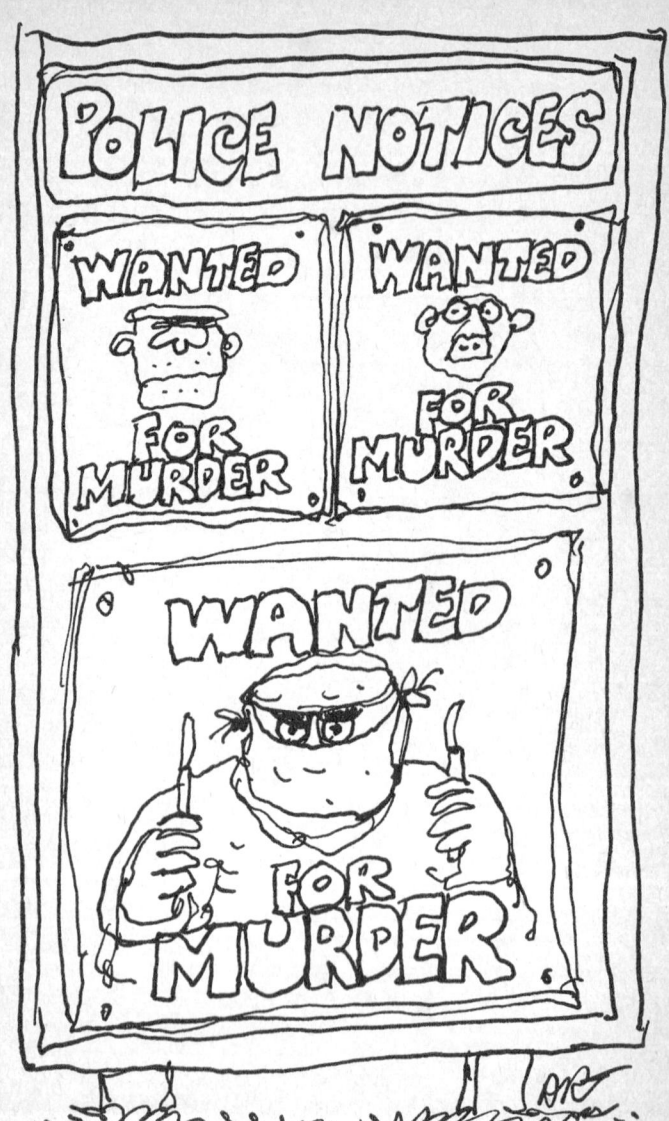

Surgeon (gravely): Before we begin, Mr Whitesides, I feel it is only right to warn you that of all the people who have undertaken this operation, statistics show that four out of every five have died.

Whitesides: Mmmm . . .

Surgeon: Now is there anything I can do for you?

Whitesides: I'll say there is! Help me on with my clothes and call a taxi, will you?

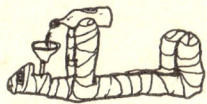

Patient: What exactly are my chances of recovery from this operation?

Surgeon: Excellent! Excellent! In fact, Mr Prone they are one hundred per cent!

Patient: But that's marvellous!

Surgeon: Yes, indeed! Statistics show that nine out of every ten die from it.

Patient: So how are my chances so wonderful?

Surgeon: Nine of my patients have already *died!* You're the *tenth!*

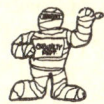

Maternity

or,

There's one born every minute!

Seen in the Ladies' Toilet in the Maternity Wing, an inspired piece of feminine thinking written on the wall saying, 'The girls of today are the mothers of tomorrow!'

Underneath this was written the profound postscript, 'So soon?'

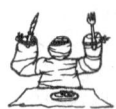

It was a solemn occasion. The Doctor delivered the baby, held him upside down in the time-honoured fashion and slapped its bottom.

The baby laughed! The Doctor looked at the midwife who looked at the Doctor, then they both looked closely at the baby and saw that one of its little fists was clenched.

Very carefully the Doctor prised open the fist, and in the middle of the baby's palm was the reason for the laughter – a little pill!

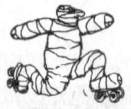

The haughty mother of the pretty girl sitting in bed in the Maternity Ward holding her new-born infant in her arms was not amused!

She stared at her daughter with complete disdain.

'Really,' she snapped, 'a mother at your age! Honestly, Vera – what got *into* you?'

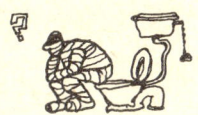

The attractive lady hailed a cab, urgently.

'The Maternity Hospital and hurry,' she cried.

The cab jerked forward as the cabbie released the brake and put his foot down.

'Don't worry,' yelled the lady from the floor. 'I only work there!'

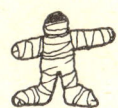

The nurse emerged holding a cute little brown baby in her arms.

The four expectant fathers waiting there for news sat up in their chairs as she approached them.

'There you are, Mr Standfast,' she crooned. 'He's all yours. Isn't he a beautiful little chap?'

Mr Standfast shook his head doubtfully at the colour.

'No,' he said, 'he's not mine. I think you've made a mistake, Nurse, he's definitely not mine... although hang about, he *could* be! My wife burns every ruddy thing!'

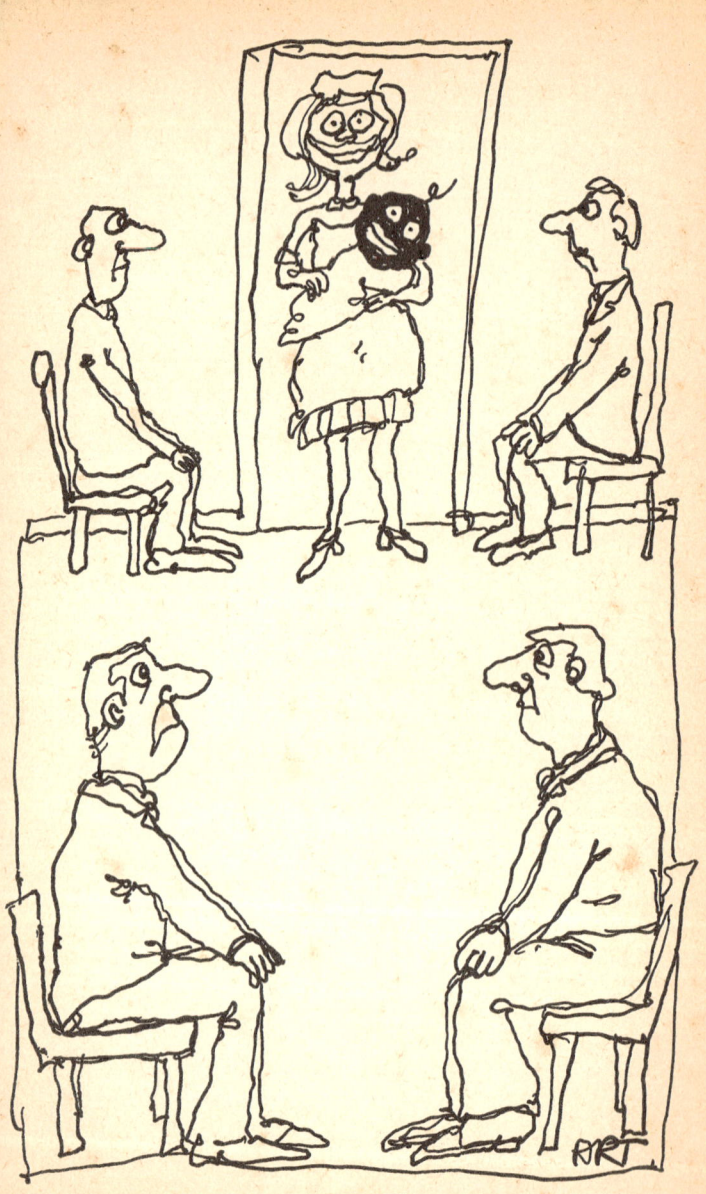

The same Nurse also emerged half-an-hour later, holding three bouncing baby girls in her arms. She went up to a happy husband who had been celebrating rather too much for the occasion.

'There you are, Mr Curtis,' she smiled. 'What d'you think of these?'

'Wonderful,' he laughed. 'I'll have the one in the middle!'

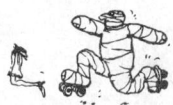

A few beds along from Vera, another pretty girl sat in bed holding her baby in her arms, crying bitterly, her boyfriend by her side.

'I've had enough, Fred,' she sobbed. 'If this is what an engagement's like I'm *never* going to get married!'

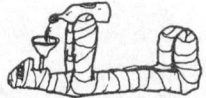

The visiting mother and father stared proudly at their daughter's baby son lying in her arms, gurgling happily away.

'Isn't he adorable?' said the mother. 'He's *so* happy!'

'Well,' said her daughter doubtfully, 'he *seems* to be happy, but I think he must cry all night, because when I woke up this morning, his crib was full of tears!'

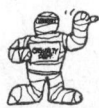

Some girls shrink from having babies.

Others get bigger and bigger . . .

Then there was the premature baby – his father wasn't expecting him!

A large notice pinned up in a Maternity Ward read as follows:
   'There are five reasons why Mother's Milk is better than Cow's Milk.
   1. It's more sanitary.
   2. It's fresher.
   3. It's easier to take to a picnic.
   4. Cats can't get at it.
   5. It comes in such *gorgeous* containers!'

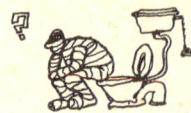

The smiling nurse came out holding three bouncing, wailing babies in her arms.
   'Mr Powell,' she called. 'Mr Powell?'
   Mr Powell jumped to his feet happily. 'I'm Powell, Nurse,' he said. 'Is it a boy?'
   She laughed. 'The one in the middle is!'

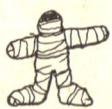

Another notice pinned up in a Maternity Ward read as follows:
   'This week is National Baby Week, and here is a message for babies all over the world: 'Kitchy-kitchy-kitchy-koo, then . . .'

A sign in a Maternity Home: *Children should be seen and not had!*

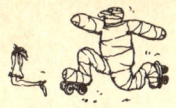

Mother 1: Well, my hubby said, 'Really, Flickers, I don't know why you want another child so quickly, we've already *got* six!' Well, I told him, I said I've always wanted children young . . .
Mother 2: I agree, dear. Who wants old children?

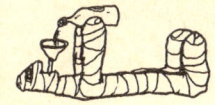

Medical Meanderings

or,

Did you know that . . . ?

If you took all the blood vessels, arteries and veins from a man and laid them side by side on the floor – that man would die!

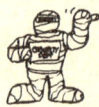

The wife of an Oil Tycoon once sent a card to her husband who was in hospital. The card said, *'Get Well Soon!'*

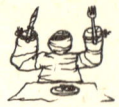

There was a Doctor who was an ear, nose and throat specialist and a bit of a tit man as well!

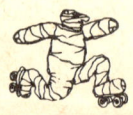

The Chief Ophthalmic Surgeon of a Hospital was retiring after many years service. As a retirement present, the Hospital asked a famous portrait painter to paint the Surgeon's portrait, and planned to present it to the Surgeon at his retirement lunch.

The important day came along, and the portrait stood proudly on an easel, covered by a white sheet ready for its unveiling.

At a given time, the string was pulled, the white sheet came away, and the painting was revealed. It was indeed a magnificent effort!

Covering the canvas was a large eye, and in the very centre of the eye, plumb in the middle of the pupil was the portrait of the Surgeon!

There was a dead silence as the Surgeon stood back admiring the portrait, but he said nothing.

Finally, a lone voice broke the silence. 'Well,' it said, 'what do you think of it?'

The Surgeon smiled.

'Thank God I'm not a Gynaecologist!' he said.

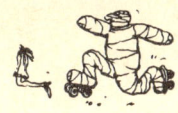

Out of penicillin you can make a mouldy green fungus?

*

The Labour Party have found a cure for influenza? They're going to nationalize it!

*

A certain Indian lady Doctor sat up all night with a Sikh friend?

*

There was a chemist's shop which was always empty? It could have been the result of their proud notice in the window which said, *'We dispense with accuracy!'*

*

There is a Plastic Surgeon treating patients in the Stockbroker belt of Weybridge, Surrey? He doesn't lift faces, he lifts noses!

*

There were two mice living in a local Health Centre. One day, they were sitting on either side of a hole in a skirting board in the Doctor's office, when in walked a ravishing blonde.

One of the mice gasped in admiration. 'Great Heavens, Stanton,' he exclaimed, 'isn't she fantastic? What about those gorgeous legs!'

'Not for me, Wayne,' said the other. 'I'm a titmouse!'

*

There is a Mail Order psychiatrist? You just tear off the top of your head and mail it to him!

*

There is a book published as a guide for those who want to know what to do until the Doctor arrives? It's called *How to make love to the Doctor's receptionist*!

*

'Alice' was something that Christopher Robin went down with!

*

All 'Do-It-Themselves' Hypochondriacs are the same — they want to have their ache and treat it!

*

There was one hypochondriac who left instructions in his will that he was to be buried by the side of his Doctor!

*

There is another hypochondriac who always treats himself from do-it-yourself medical books. It is feared that one day he will die from a misprint!

*

A million germs can live on the point of a needle? What a stupid diet!

*

The trouble with child psychology is that the parents understand it, but the kids don't!

*

If all the people who go to consult a psychiatrist were laid end-to-end – it would take an extremely large couch!

*

They say that One Pound notes carry germs? Ridiculous! Even a germ can't live on a quid these days!

*

Two 'flu germs met on a handkerchief? One said, 'Hi, George, how are things?' George said, 'Not so good, Hedley. I think I'm going down with a touch of penicillin!'

*

Dick Turpin was the first man to save beds for the National Health with his policy of 'Stand and Deliver!'

*

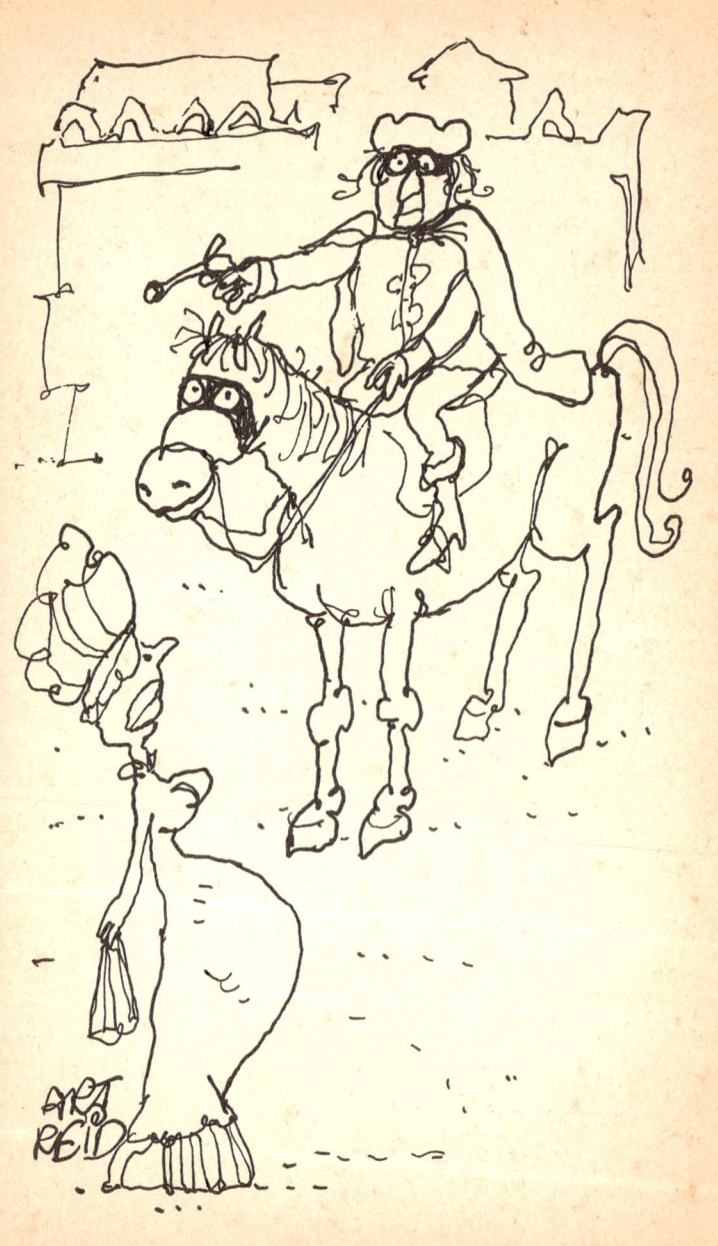

Two students of an Anatomy Lecture were bored with the very uninteresting skeletons hanging around, mainly because the most interesting bits were missing. This they couldn't understand, until the girl student suddenly hit on the answer as to why they *were* missing. Obviously, the best bits didn't have bones in them!

*

If a fat man and a thin man are cremated at the same time, which one turns to ashes first? Neither: it's a dead heat.

*

Did you know that Davy Crockett had three ears? One on the left, one on the right . . . and a wild frontier.

Around the wards

or,

Hospital glaze

There was a male patient in one ward who fancied a certain nurse so much she had to hold his wrist to check his *im*pulse!

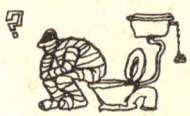

'Oh Doctor,' the patient moaned during Doctor's Rounds, 'every time I lift my arm an agonizing pain shoots right down it.'
   'So don't lift it!'

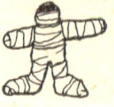

One patient was given so many different coloured sleeping pills, he had dreams in technicolour!

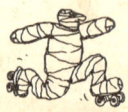

The once-handsome man felt his strength seeping slowly and finally from him, as he lay on his hospital bed, his wife leaning silently and attentively over him to catch his every faint word.

He felt guilt welling up inside him as he gazed at her gentle, loving face watching his life slip away. He had to tell her. It was only right that she should know what a cad he had been.

'Darling,' he whispered. 'No! Please don't stop me. I – I must tell you ... now ... before it's too late. Darling, I've been a cad – yes, and a rotter! I – I've been unfaithful to you.'

He paused to allow his words to sink in.

'You know I was supposed to have those late company meetings on Tuesday and Friday nights?' She nodded. He continued, 'I didn't. I was making love to Stephanie Fullbody! And you know those weekends I was supposed to be away in Manchester with our branch contact, Phil Burns?' She nodded. He continued, 'I wasn't! I was making love to Felicity Curvey. And – and you know I was supposed to be working late at the office on Mondays, Wednesdays and Thursdays?' Again she nodded. Again he continued, 'Well, I wasn't! I was making love to Daphne Titley.'

He fell back on his pillow, exhausted. 'My conscience is now clear,' he breathed. 'I – I wanted you to know.'

'I already did, darling,' she said softly. 'Who d'you think gave you the poison?'

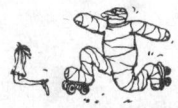

There was the patient who hated being sent for X-Rays, but he had to grin and barium!

Two ladies in adjoining beds had just woken up.

1st Lady: Oh! What a *dreadful* dream I've just had! Oh! It was *so* embarrassing!

2nd Lady: Really? What was it all about?

1st Lady: Well, I went to this wedding, all dressed up – as I thought – but instead, there was I, yours truly, walking down the aisle in my birthday suit!

2nd Lady: My word.

1st Lady: Mine, too! There I was – nothing on except a *hat*! I was absolutely humiliated!

2nd Lady: Why, dear?

1st Lady: It was last year's hat!

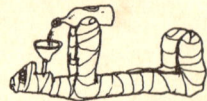

Then there was the ex-seaman who was so sick that the ship tattooed on his chest was lowering life-boats!

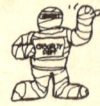

One patient nipped out to the ward loo so often, the others nick-named him Flush Gordon!

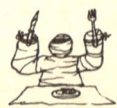

Male Patient: Nurse, could I have some orange juice, please?

Nurse: Certainly, Mr Russell. I'll give you some with pleasure.

Patient: Oh! Perks, already!

The Casanova of the ward was chatting up his favourite Nurse, with sweet words of love.

'We'll have a wonderful life together,' he murmured, softly. 'The home you've always dreamed about, roses around the front door, a lovely garden, we'll build our own nursery, listen to the patter of tiny feet, and one day . . . one day, who knows? We might even get married!'

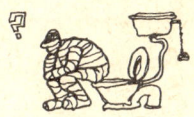

Mr Greenough: Here, Nurse! Give us a kiss!
Nurse (indignant): No!
Mr Greenough: Come on. You *know* you will, in the end.
Nurse: Oh? Who said I would?
Mr Greenough: Everybody!

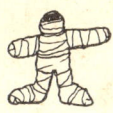

Patient (to visitor): Oh, they're marvellous in this ward. They're always around with tea. They say it keeps us going.
Visitor: Yes – and I'll bet I know where!

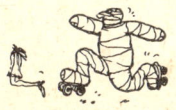

One of the patients was a wealthy playboy suffering from High Blonde Pressure!

The Casanova was at it again.

'Nurse,' he whispered, 'when the lights go out, what about popping into bed with me?'

The Nurse was horrified. 'Do you mind?' she snapped. 'I'm not like that! Besides, my mother says there are certain things a girl should just not do before twenty-one!'

The Casanova nodded thoughtfully.

'I suppose she's right! I hate an audience!'

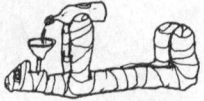

Then there was the politician who was taken in, suffering from a mental hernia!

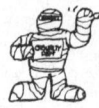

One patient was so vain he wanted his X-Rays retouched!

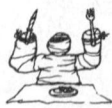

Mr Hoggitt was having his pre-med jab before the operation.

As the Nurse bent over him, he sobbed, 'They can't let me die, Nurse! They *mustn't* let me die! I'm the father of fourteen children!'

'Well done, Mr Hoggitt,' said the nurse, 'but this is no time to brag!'

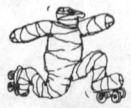

One of the patients had a marvellous dream one night. He dreamed he was eating a giant marshmallow. He loved marshmallows so he enjoyed his outsized meal although it seemed to go on forever.

Finally he finished it and, licking his lips and wishing there was some more of it left for tomorrow night, he resumed an uninterrupted night's sleep.

When he woke up in the morning he found his pillow was gone!

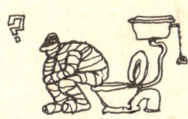

The rugby player in bed six was in a bad way, and the Doctor wanted to know how it all happened.

'Well,' said the player, 'I was playing at outside half. The ball came back very slowly, and as I picked it up, these two flank forwards grabbed me. Each of them took hold of one of my legs, and the last thing I remember is one of them saying to the other, "Make a wish!" '

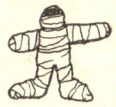

There was the patient who took a turn for the Nurse!

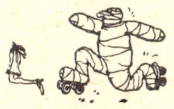

'What happened to old Campbell in bed seven?'
'They moved him – said he was too ugly for wards!'

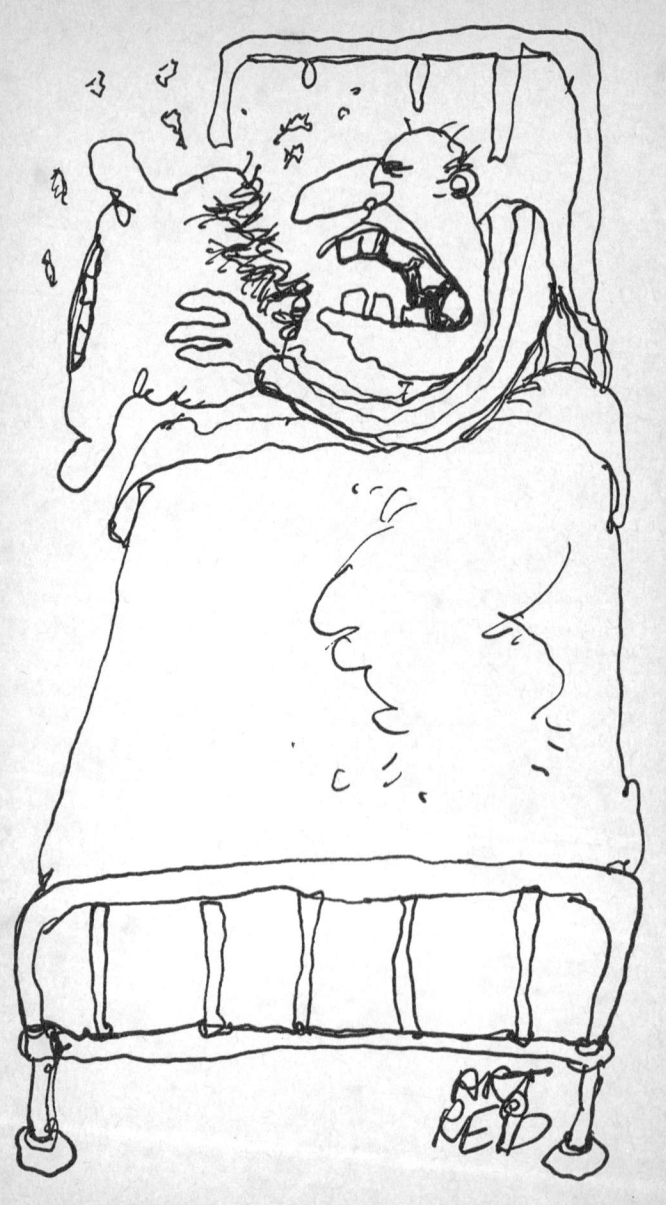

Queen Victoria was visiting the sick in a hospital during World War I. There were three soldiers in the ward. She asked the first, 'What's wrong with you?'

'Diarrhoea, Your Majesty,' he replied.

'And what is your greatest wish?'

'To get well soon and to get back to the fighting.'

She turned to the doctor and asked him what they were doing to cure the man.

He said, 'We give him a wire brush, dip it in ointment and he brushes this on the affected parts.'

She walked over to the second man and asked him his complaint.

'Piles, Your Majesty.'

Again she asked him what his greatest wish was and he replied, 'To get back to the front again once I'm better.'

Again, she turned to the doctor and asked how they're helping the man recover.

The doctor replied as before: 'We give him a wire brush dipped in ointment and he spreads this on the affected parts.'

At the end of the ward was the third man and Queen Victoria went up to him.

'And what is wrong with you?'

'Mouth ulcers, Your Majesty,' he said.

'And what is your greatest wish?'

'To get the brush before the other two!'

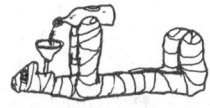

A gynaecologist came home from a hard day's work, to be greeted by his wife at the front door . . . 'Hello dear, had a nice day at the orifice?'

A man was very seriously injured in an accident, so much so that the only part left whole was his head. He'd been in hospital some time when Christmas came and his mother came to give him a present.

'Here,' she said, 'something to cheer you up, I've brought you a Christmas present.'

He opened it and said, 'Oh no, not another bloody hat!'

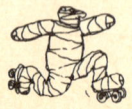

Dear Doctor . . .

or,

Don't call me and I won't call you!

Dear Doctor . . .

Is kleptomania catching?
No! It's taking!

*

What causes water on the knee?
A tap on the head!

*

What can I do for a hangover?
Simple, Madam. Wear a larger bra!

*

How can I avoid falling hair?
Jump out of the way!

*

Is hay-fever positive or negative?
Both! Sometimes the 'eyes' have it, and sometimes the 'nose'!

*

What is the cause of baldness?
Too much skin!

*

I can't sleep at nights. Can you suggest a cure?
Certainly. Move over to the edge of the bed – you'll soon drop off!

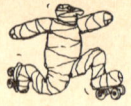

NB:
THERE IS NO APPENDIX IN THIS BOOK — IT HAS BEEN REMOVED!

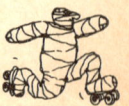

All Futura Books are available at your bookshop or newsagent, or can be ordered from the following address:
Futura Books, Cash Sales Department,
P.O. Box 11, Falmouth, Cornwall.

Please send cheque or postal order (no currency), and allow 45p for postage and packing for the first book plus 20p for the second book and 14p for each additional book ordered up to a maximum charge of £1.63 in U.K.

Customers in Eire and B.F.P.O. please allow 45p for the first book, 20p for the second book plus 14p per copy for the next 7 books, thereafter 8p per book.

Overseas customers please allow 75p for postage and packing for the first book and 21p per copy for each additional book.

JOKE BOOKS

If you're an eager Beaver reader, perhaps you ought to try some more of our hilarious Beaver joke books. They are available in bookshops or they can be ordered directly from us. Just complete the form below and enclose the right amount of money and the books will be sent to you at home.

☐	THE BROWNIE JOKE BOOK	Brownies	95p
☐	MORE BROWNIE JOKES	Brownies	95p
☐	JELLYBONE GRAFFITI BOOK	Therese Birch	95p
☐	SCHOOL GRAFFITI	Peter Eldin	95p
☐	SKOOL FOR LAUGHS	Peter Eldin	95p
☐	THE WOOLLY JUMPER JOKE BOOK	Peter Eldin	95p
☐	THE FUNNIEST JOKE BOOK	Jim Eldridge	£1.00
☐	THE WOBBLY JELLY JOKE BOOK	Jim Eldridge	95p
☐	HOW TO HANDLE GROWN-UPS	Jim Eldridge	£1.00
☐	THE CRAZY JOKER'S HANDBOOK	Janet Rogers	£1.00
☐	THE CRAZY JOKE BOOK STRIKES BACK	Janet Rogers	£1.00
☐	THE ELEPHANT JOKE BOOK	Katie Wales	£1.00
☐	FALL ABOUT WITH FLO	Floella Benjamin	£1.25

And if you would like to hear more about Beaver Books, and find out all the latest news, don't forget the BEAVER BULLETIN. Just send a stamped, self-addressed envelope to Beaver Books, 62 – 65 Chandos Place, Covent Garden, London WC2N 4NW.

If you would like to order books, please send this form, and the money due to:

HAMLYN PAPERBACK CASH SALES, PO BOX 11, FALMOUTH, CORNWALL TR10 9EN.

Send a cheque or postal order, and don't forget to include postage at the following rates: UK: 55p for first book, 22p for the second, 14p thereafter; BFPO and Eire: 55p for first book, 22p for the second, 14p per copy for next 7 books, 8p per book thereafter; Overseas £1.00 for first book, 25p thereafter.

NAME..

ADDRESS...

....

Please print clearly

THE ELEPHANT JOKE BOOK

Katie Wales

What do you get if you cross an elephant with a biscuit?
Crumbs!

How can you tell if you have an elephant in bed with you?
By the 'E' embroidered on his pyjamas!

How do you catch an elephant?
Make a noise like a peanut.

You'll find tons of fun, giggles and groans in this jumbo collection of jokes, riddles and rhymes about elephants of every shape, size and colour. An enormous book full of tall stories and elephant jokes that you'll never forget . . .

FALL ABOUT WITH FLO

Floella Benjamin

Between the pages of this book, Floella Benjamin, regular presenter of TV's 'Playschool' invites you to have a good laugh with her over some of the funniest jokes you've ever heard. Come along and join the fun!

What's green and hard?
A frog with a machine gun.

Doctor, doctor, I think I'm a billiard ball!
Get to the end of the queue.

What did the sofa say to the painting?
You're up the wall.

What did the car say to the road sign?
You're round the bend.

What did the astronaut say to mission control?
I'm over the moon.

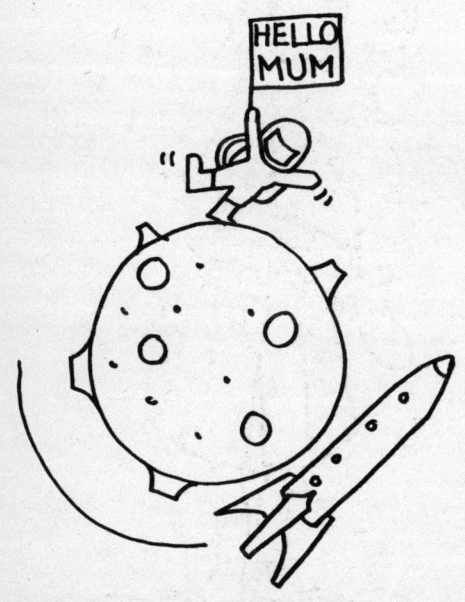

What did the doll say to the broken rocking-
  horse?
You're off your rocker.

WALLY: *The teacher likes me more than you.*
ERIC: How do you know?
WALLY: *She puts more kisses on my homework
  than yours.*

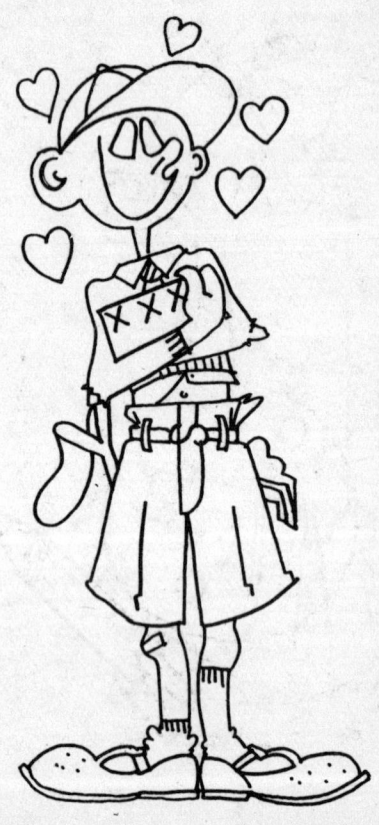

'Dad, do slugs taste nice?'
'Why do you ask, son?'
''Cos you've just eaten the one that was in your salad!'

'Hey, Wally's found a job with plenty of openings.'
'What is it?'
'A doorman at the Grand Hotel.'

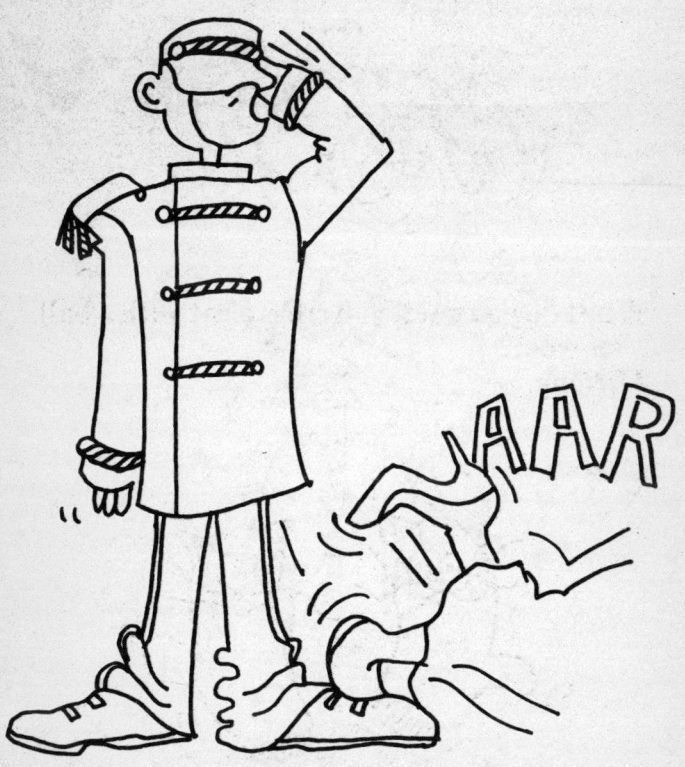

'Doctor! Doctor! I feel like a piece of a jigsaw!'
'OK I'll fit you in later.'

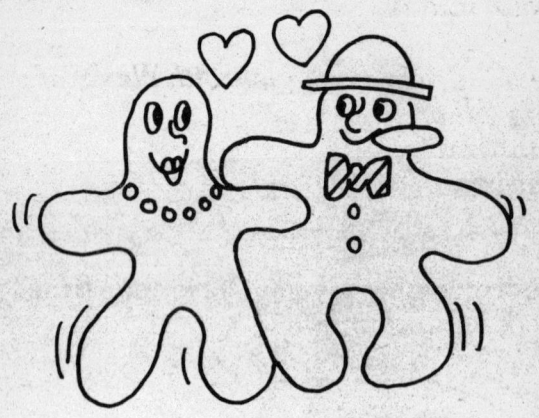

What do you get if you cross a cat with a ball of wool?
Mittens.

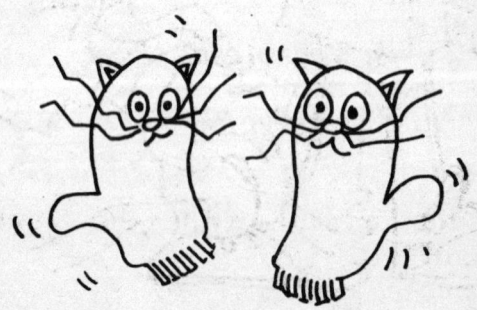

What did the little clock hand say to the big clock hand?
See you in an hour.

'How did you break your leg, Wally?'
'Tim fell on it.'
'Tim who?'
'Timber.'

Where do ghosts go at Christmas time?
To the phantomime.

'Doctor! Doctor! I feel like a telephone!'
Well don't get hung up about it.'

'Doctor! Doctor! I feel like a computer!'
'Right, let's get down to basics.'

WALLY: *I'd like a bar of soap please.*
SHOP ASSISTANT: Scented?
WALLY: *No, I'll take it with me.*

What did the vicar say when the church caught fire?
Holy smoke!